The Comprehensive DIABETIC COOKBOOK

Dorothy Kaplan

With a Foreword by Robert Kaye, M.D., Professor and Chairman, Department of Pediatrics, Hahnemann Medical College and Hospital, Philadelphia, and Board Member, the American Diabetes Association

Every person who plans meals for a diabetic contends with the complex formulas of the Diabetic Exchange Diet. The exchange values in a meat, potato, and vegetable menu are simple enough to determine, but how does one calculate the exchanges in a more exotic mixed dish such as Chili Con Carne?

Easy-to-prepare recipes provide the meal-planning answers in *The Comprehensive Diabetic Cookbook.* This completely revised and updated manual enables diabetics to enjoy an extensive and varied diet without sacrificing accurate control of exchanges, calories, and food composition. Each recipe is broken down into food exchange values, as well as calorie, protein, carbohydrate, and fat compositions—information that is equally important to non-diabetics who wish to keep a strict eye on calorie or cholesterol intake. Now the diabetic can dine on delectable culinary classics such as Bouillabaisse, Chicken Paella,

(Continued on back flap)

Hospital, Philadelphia, Pennsylvania. He is also a member of the board of the American Diabetes Association.

THE COMPREHENSIVE
DIABETIC COOKBOOK

THE COMPREHENSIVE DIABETIC COOKBOOK

Completely Revised and Updated

by

DOROTHY J. KAPLAN

WITH A FOREWORD BY
Robert Kaye, M.D.,
Professor and Chairman, Department of Pediatrics,
Hahnemann Medical College and Hospital, Philadelphia
and Board Member, American Diabetes Association

GREENWICH HOUSE
Distributed by Crown Publishers, Inc.
New York

To my husband, Jerry, who is everything.

Copyright © MCMLXXII, MCMLXXXI by Dorothy J. Kaplan

All rights reserved.

This 1984 edition is published by Greenwich House,
a division of Arlington House, Inc.,
distributed by Crown Publishers, Inc.,
by arrangement with Frederick Fell Publishers, Inc.

Manufactured in the United States of America

Library of Congress Cataloging in Publication Data

Kaplan, Dorothy J.
. The comprehensive diabetic cookbook.

Bibliography: p.
includes index.
1. Diabetes—Diet therapy—Recipes. I. Title.
RC662.K36 1984   641.5′6314   82-83772
ISBN: 0-517-444534
h g f e d c b a

Contents

Foreword

Mrs. Kaplan has very successfully managed all aspects of diabetic regulation since her daughter became diabetic at the age of two years.

I believe that her manual offers a great deal which will be useful to other diabetics and to individuals interested in controlling or reducing their weight. The scope of the manual is so extensive that the user will be enabled to enjoy a widely varied diet without sacrificing accurate control of calories and composition. Presentation of individual food items in terms of calories, protein, carbohydrate, and fat composition as well as in the exchange system is particularly helpful to users who may be familiar with only one or the other system of calculation.

In addition, the manual will be a valuable adjunct to the doctor and will satisfy a need which I have long felt in my practice with reference to children with diabetes and obesity. I, for one, am grateful to Mrs. Kaplan for having taken the great pains to bring this comprehensive book to completion.

ROBERT KAYE, M.D.
Professor and Chairman
Department of Pediatrics
Hahnemann Medical College and
Hospital, Philadelphia

Introduction

Since our daughter developed diabetes, I have spent a great deal of time calculating and revising our favorite recipes, developing new ones, and writing to companies to acquire carbohydrate, protein, and fat breakdowns of their products. Having this information greatly simplified my menu planning. As the diabetic diet is a natural, well-balanced one, I preferred making the same dishes for the entire family to cooking two separate meals three times a day. It was a challenge to make our meals interesting, varied, and delicious.

The result of this research and investigation was the compilation of this "manual." And once it took shape, grew, and I began using it, I realized how handy and timesaving it was. I hope that other diabetics, those cooking for diabetics, and those interested in wholesome, tasty recipes will find it of help.

The diabetic's diet must be carefully balanced in carbohydrates, proteins, and fat; the exchange system enables this balance to be maintained easily. Your physician will work out your menus by calculating how many exchanges you are allowed per meal in every category. Using this manual you can then plan varied and delicious meals. Suppose he tells you your breakfast should consist of:

1 fruit exchange
1½ bread exchanges
2 medium-fat meat exchanges
½ milk exchange
1 fat exchange

Turning to the fruit section of this manual you can see that you might have ½ cup orange juice *or* 1 orange *or* 1 peach *or* ½ banana *or* any other listing under fruit exchange. Your 1½ bread exchanges might be ¾ cup dry cereal (1 bread exchange)

ix

and ½ piece toast (½ bread exchange) or 1½ pieces toast (1½ bread exchanges) or 1½ muffins (1½ bread exchanges) or any other total of 1½ under the bread exchange. Your 2 medium-fat meat exchanges could be 2 scrambled eggs (or poached or soft boiled, etc.) or 2 ounces of medium-fat meat. The ½ milk exchange, which would be 4 ounces of skim milk, could be used in your cereal. The one fat exchange could be a slice of bacon to go with your eggs or 1 teaspoon butter or margarine to go on your toast.

If your diet is set up in calories, rather than exchanges, follow the same procedure using the calorie listing under each exchange:

1 milk exchange—80 calories
1 vegetable exchange—25 calories
1 fruit exchange—40 calories
1 bread exchange—70 calories
1 low-fat meat exchange—55 calories
1 fat exchange—45 calories

Many diabetics have followed this system for years but were unable to eat anything other than those foods listed in each exchange category. They were not able to eat a mixed food, such as meat loaf or potato salad or chicken cacciatora or any recipe that called for a combination of ingredients because they couldn't figure out how much of each exchange the serving of food would provide. Here we provide the answer to this problem. Every recipe in this book lists the exchanges that a serving will provide. If you have a serving of potato salad in Chapter 5, you will know that you are consuming one bread exchange and four fat exchanges. One serving of ribbon meat loaf in Chapter 9 will provide you with three high-fat meat exchanges, one bread exchange and one fat exchange. You can see immediately how much of each dish the diabetic may eat using the diet outlined by your physician. Everyone will benefit; the diabetic will eat tasty dishes and the rest of the family will eat the well-balanced meals on which all diabetic diets are based.

Thus, you can see the value and outstanding merit of this system. There is great variety of meal-planning and ease of cooking because the exchange system and these recipes are based on handy household measures. In addition, after you have become familiar with these recipes, you can turn to the appendix and, using the forms provided, calculate your own favorite dishes.

The emphasis on dietary control of diabetes is being stressed more today than ever before, and a proper diet that is tasty and easy to follow is as important as the medication prescribed. My sincere hope is that the recipes in this book will make it easier for you to follow the proper diet, and that this will add happy and healthy years to your life.

DJK

To Those Watching Their Weight

There are very few people who haven't tried a "fad" or "crash" diet once or twice, knowing that the real answer to losing weight and maintaining the proper scale-reading is sensible, well-balanced, controlled eating. The diabetic formula can easily be adapted by the normal weight watcher.

The first step is a visit to your physician. After a checkup and discussion as to your weight requirements, he will work out for you a diet based on exchanges; you will know how much of each exchange you are allowed per meal and thus, using his list and this manual as a guide, you can plan your daily meals. They will be adequate, varied, interesting, and calculated for you, so your eating program will be well-balanced and you will be on your way to your proper weight.

For instance, let us say your doctor prescribes the following 1500-calorie-per-day diet for you:

Breakfast

1 fruit exchange
1 low-fat meat exchange
1 bread exchange
1 fat exchange
½ milk exchange

Lunch

3 low-fat meat exchanges
1 vegetable exchange
1½ bread exchanges
2 fat exchanges
1 fruit exchange
½ milk exchange

Dinner

3 low-fat meat exchanges
1 vegetable exchange
1 bread exchange
1 fat exchange
1 fruit exchange
½ milk exchange

Snack

½ milk exchange
1 bread exchange

Using the exchange lists at the head of each of the seven categories—milk, fat, vegetable, fruit, bread, meat—and adding the calculated recipes in this manual, you can plan countless different meals. For dinner you could have:

Egg drop soup
Flank steak
Pseudo sweet-potato casserole
Gelatin and fruit salad
1 apple muffin
Jellied blanc mange

OR

Shish kabob
¼ cup beets
Orange marmalade nut bread
½ cup applesauce
Pudding surprise

OR

Tomato tantalizer
Barbecued chuck roast
Baked potato
Broccoli
Parfait royale

As you can see, the possibilities are endless and the results truly delicious.

In planning a meal, list the exchanges allowed for that meal. Then, as you select a recipe and see what exchanges will be used in a serving, cross out those exchanges on your list. In that manner you can see what you have left as you go along. Be sure to carefully measure each serving.

Following this system is like playing a game; you will come up with different, delicious meals all the time and you won't believe you're weight-watching!

A Special Note Regarding "Dietetic" or "Sugar-Free" Packaged Foods

It is most important to realize that all foods must be calculated in the diet. If something says "dietetic" or "sugar-free," is still has calories and must be counted. Most of these special foods have a substance substituted for sugar and it is stated that this substance is utilized by the body at a much slower rate than sugar would be utilized. This is true, but since the substance is utilized by the body, the calories must be subtracted from the daily allowance.

All such special products state the caloric content on the container. It is wise to compare the calories in the artificially sweetened product with the real thing. Often the difference is negligible and the dietetic or sugar-free product does not usually taste as good. If you have to count the calories anyway, why not enjoy the better flavor.

THE COMPREHENSIVE
DIABETIC COOKBOOK

CHAPTER 1

Milk

MILK EXCHANGES

One milk exchange consists of:

Carbohydrate	12 grams
Protein	8 grams
Fat	Trace
Calories	80

This list shows the kinds and amounts of milk or milk products to use for one milk exchange. Those which appear in **bold type** are **non-fat.** Low-fat and whole milk contain saturated fat.

Non-Fat Fortified Milk
Skim or non-fat milk   1 cup
Powdered (non-fat dry, before adding liquid)   ⅓ cup
Canned, evaporated—skim milk   ½ cup
Buttermilk made from skim milk   1 cup
Yogurt made from skim milk (plain, unflavored) 1 cup

Low-Fat Fortified Milk
1% fat fortified milk   1 cup
   (omit ½ fat exchange)
2% fat fortified milk   1 cup
   (omit 1 fat exchange)
Yogurt made from 2% fortified milk
   (plain, unflavored)   1 cup
   (omit 1 fat exchange)

Whole Milk (Omit 2 fat exchanges)
    Whole milk   1 cup
    Canned, evaporated whole milk   ½ cup
    Buttermilk made from whole milk   1 cup
    Yogurt made from whole milk (plain,
        unflavored)   1 cup

Dessert and beverage recipes sometimes provide milk exchanges. If you will refer to Chapter 16 you will find the following recipes can be figured in your diet as milk exchanges:

Cherry-Cream Pie Filling
Baked Custard
Jellied Blanc Mange
Baked Alaska
Pudding Surprise
Parfait Royale

In Chapter 19, Beverages, you will find a recipe for milkshakes that is calculated in milk exchanges.

CHAPTER 2

Fat Exchanges

FAT EXCHANGES

One fat exchange consists of:

Fat	5 grams
Calories	45

This list shows the kinds and amounts of fat-containing foods to use for one fat exchange. To plan a diet low in saturated fat select only those exchanges which appear in **bold type.** They are **polyunsaturated.**

Margarine, soft, tub or stick*	1 teaspoon
Avocado (4″ in diameter)**	⅛
Oil, corn, cottonseed, safflower, soy, sunflower	1 teaspoon
Oil, olive**	1 teaspoon
Oil, peanut**	1 teaspoon
Olives**	5 small
Almonds**	10 whole
Pecans**	2 large whole
Peanuts**	
Spanish	20 whole
Virginia	10 whole
Walnuts	6 small
Nuts, other**	6 small

*Made with corn, cottonseed, safflower, soy or sunflower oil only
**Fat content is primarily monounsaturated

3

Margarine, regular stick	1 teaspoon
Butter	1 teaspoon
Bacon fat	1 teaspoon
Bacon, crisp	1 strip
Cream, light	2 tablespoons
Cream, sour	2 tablespoons
Cream, heavy	1 tablespoon
Cream cheese	1 tablespoon
French dressing***	1 tablespoon
Italian dressing***	1 tablespoon
Lard	1 teaspoon
Mayonnaise***	1 teaspoon
Salad dressing, mayonnaise type***	2 teaspoons
Salt pork	¾ inch cube

***If made with corn, cottonseed, safflower, soy or sunflower oil can be used on fat modified diet

CHAPTER 3

Vegetable Exchanges and Recipes

VEGETABLE EXCHANGES

One vegetable exchange consists of:

Carbohydrates	5 grams
Protein	2 grams
Calories	25

This list shows the kinds of **vegetables** to use for one vegetable exchange. One exchange is ½ cup.

Asparagus
Bean Sprouts
Beets
Broccoli
Brussels Sprouts
Cabbage
Carrots
Cauliflower
Celery
Cucumbers
Eggplant
Green Pepper
Greens:
  Beet
  Chards
  Collards
  Dandelion
  Kale
Greens:
  Mustard
  Spinach
  Turnip
Mushrooms
Okra
Onions
Rhubarb
Rutabaga
Sauerkraut
String Beans, green or
  yellow
Summer Squash
Tomatoes
Tomato Juice
Turnips
Vegetable Juice Cocktail
Zucchini

The following **raw vegetables** may be used as desired:

Chicory   Lettuce
Chinese Cabbage   Parsley
Endive   Radishes
Escarole   Watercress

Starchy Vegetables are found in the Bread Exchange List.
When cooking frozen vegetables in butter sauce, add 1 fat
exchange for each ½ cup serving.

Frozen vegetables can be baked. Place block in casserole;
spread with margarine, sprinkle with salt (for limas only, add
¼ cup water). Cover and bake along with dinner. (Be sure to
calculate margarine out of fat allowance.)

Chart is for baking at 350 degrees. If baking at 325 degrees
increase time ten minutes; if baking at 375 degrees decrease
time ten minutes.

40 to 50 minutes
   Broccoli
   Peas
   Spinach
   Squash
   Brussels sprouts
   Whole kernel corn
   Limas, large

50 to 60 minutes
   Asparagus
   Cauliflower
   Green beans
   Limas, small
   Mixed vegetables
   Peas and carrots
   Succotash

Brand-name vegetable products and their exchanges are
listed in an appendix at the back of the book.

RECIPE FOR

Fabulous Salad

Ingredients	Measure	Carbohydrates (gm.)	Protein (gm.)	Fat (gm.)
Eggplant, medium, cubed	1 cup	10	4	
Zucchini, medium, sliced	1 cup	10	4	
Green pepper, cubed	1 cup	10	4	
Tomatoes, cubed	1 cup	10	4	
Onions, sliced, large	1 cup	10	4	
Garlic, sliced	2			
Mushrooms, sliced	1 pound	20	8	
Oil	¼ cup			60
Tomato juice	½ cup	5	2	
Salt	2 teaspoons			
Pepper	½ teaspoon			
		75	30	60

Calories: 1 serving—96   75   3   6

Combine all ingredients in large baking dish, season with salt and pepper and mix well. Bake 40 minutes at 350 degrees. Stir once or twice.

Servings: 10
Exchange per serving: 1½ vegetable, 1 fat

Smothered Onions

Ingredients	Measure	Car-bohy-drates (gm.)	Pro-tein (gm.)	Fat (gm.)
Margarine	¼ cup			60
Onions, peeled and thinly sliced	10 medium	50	20	
Salt	1 teaspoon			
Pepper	⅛ teaspoon			
Worcestershire sauce	2 teaspoons			
Liquid hot pepper seasoning	dash			
		50	20	60
Calories: 1 serving—82		5	2	6

Slowly heat margarine in large skillet. Add rest of ingredients. Cook, over low heat and stirring occasionally, 30 minutes or until onions are nicely browned.

Servings: 10
Exchange per serving: 1 vegetable, 1 fat

Zing Salad

Ingredients	Measure	Carbohydrates (gm.)	Protein (gm.)	Fat (gm.)
Green beans, drained	2 cups	20	8	
Carrots, sliced and drained	2 cups	20	8	
Kidney beans, drained	2 cups	80	30	2
Onion, sliced	1 small	2.5	1	
Green pepper, chopped	¼ cup	2.5	1	
Celery, chopped	¼ cup	2.5	1	
Parsley	2 tablespoons			
White vinegar	½ cup			
Artificial sweetener	= ½ cup sugar			
Salad oil	2 tablespoons			30
Salt	1 teaspoon			
Dry mustard	1 teaspoon			
		127.5	49	32
Calories: 1 serving—95		13	5	3

Place first 7 ingredients in shallow dish. In separate container, with tight lid, place next 5 ingredients. Shake well. Pour over vegetables and refrigerate overnight.

Servings: 10
Exchange per serving: 2 vegetable, ½ fat

RECIPE FOR

Escalloped Tomatoes

Ingredients	Measure		Carbohydrates (gm.)	Protein (gm.)	Fat (gm.)
Onion, chopped	4	tablespoons	2.5	1	
Margarine, melted	1	tablespoon			15
Tomatoes	2	16-ounce cans	40	16	
Artificial sweetener	= ½	teaspoon sugar			
Salt	¾	teaspoon			
Pepper	½	teaspoon			
Soft bread crumbs, toasted	1½	cups	45	6	
			87.5	23	15
Calories: 1 serving—148			22	6	4

Sauté onion in margarine until tender. Add tomatoes, artificial sweetener, salt, and pepper; turn into 1-quart casserole. Top with bread crumbs. Bake at 375 degrees for 20 minutes. Stir lightly and serve.

Servings: 4
Exchange per serving: ¾ bread, 2 vegetable, 1 fat

Tomatoes Provencal

Ingredients	Measure	Carbohydrates (gm.)	Protein (gm.)	Fat (gm.)
Tomatoes	6 large	22.5	9	
Salt	as desired			
Pepper	as desired			
Fresh bread crumbs	1 cup	30	4	
Finely chopped parsley	2 tablespoons			
Olive oil	1 teaspoon			5
		52.5	13	5

Calories: 1 serving—53   9   2   1

Wash tomatoes and cut in half, crosswise. Place halves, cut side up, in shallow baking pan. Sprinkle each lightly with salt and pepper. Combine bread crumbs and parsley. Sprinkle over surface of tomato halves. Sprinkle each lightly with olive oil; bake at 450 degrees for 10 to 15 minutes or until golden brown on top.

Servings: 6
Exchange per serving: ½ bread, ½ vegetable

Pickles

Ingredients	Measure	Car-bohy-drates (gm.)	Pro-tein (gm.)	Fat (gm.)
Small, hard pickling cucumbers	½ bushel			
Salt	1 tablespoon per jar			
Garlic, diced	1 clove per jar			
Pickling spice	¼ teaspoon per jar			
Dill flower	2 per jar			

Scrub cucumbers with sponge or brush. Pack tightly in clean quart jars. Add remaining ingredients. Fill each jar to top with cold water. Use two-piece metal tops; boil tops and put on jars when hot; tighten and turn upside down for 24 hours. Check for leakage. Turn right side up and store in cool dark place. Ready in approximately 3 weeks. Will keep indefinitely until opened.

Can pickle tomatoes the same way by substituting hard, green tomatoes for the pickles and one half stalk celery for the two dill flowers.

Yield: 20 to 24 jars
Exchange per serving: ½ cup = 1 vegetable

Green Bean Casserole

Ingredients	Measure	Car-bohy-drates (gm.)	Pro-tein (gm.)	Fat (gm.)
Cream of chicken soup	1 10½-ounce can	20.7	9.6	17.4
Soy sauce	1 teaspoon			
French fried onion rings	3 ounces	22	3	15
French style green beans, cooked	2 1-pound cans, drained	20	8	
Pepper	dash			
		62.7	20.6	32.4
Calories: 1 serving—104		10.4	3.4	5.4

In a 1-quart casserole stir soup and soy sauce until smooth; mix in half the onions, all the beans, and the pepper. Bake at 350 degrees for 20 minutes or until bubbling. Top with remaining onions. Bake 5 minutes more.

Servings: 6
Exchange per serving: ½ bread, ½ vegetable, 1 fat

13

Carrot Pennies

Ingredients	Measure	Car-bohy-drates (gm.)	Pro-tein (gm.)	Fat (gm.)
Carrots, very thinly sliced	4 cups	20	8	
Dried basil leaves	½ teaspoon			
Salt	½ teaspoon			
Pepper	a few grains			
Water	¼ cup			
Margarine	2 tablespoons			30
		20	8	30

Calories: 1 serving—61   3   1   5

Place carrots in 1½-quart casserole. Sprinkle with basil, salt, and pepper; toss together. Add water and dot with margarine. Cover and bake at 350 degrees for 65 to 70 minutes, until fork tender.

Servings: 6
Exchange per serving: ½ vegetable, 1 fat

Pseudo Sweet-Potato Casserole

Ingredients	Measure	Carbohydrates (gm.)	Protein (gm.)	Fat (gm.)
Frozen squash, mashed	3 cups	30	12	
Artificial sweetener =	18 teaspoons sugar			
Maple flavoring, dietetic	½ teaspoon			
Dietetic orange marmalade	¼ cup			
Brown sugar	2 tablespoons	26		
Cinnamon	1 teaspoon			
Salt	1 teaspoon			
		56	12	

Calories: 1 serving—34   7   1.5

Thaw frozen squash in top of double boiler. Combine with all other ingredients. Stir until well blended. Pour into lightly oiled casserole. Bake at 350 degrees for 30 minutes.

Servings: 8
Exchange per serving: 1 vegetable

Orange Squash

Ingredients	Measure	Car-bohy-drates (gm.)	Pro-tein (gm.)	Fat (gm.)
Frozen squash, thawed	4 cups	40	16	
Margarine	¼ cup			60
Brown sugar	4 tablespoons	26		
Orange juice	¼ cup	5		
Salt	1 teaspoon			
Pepper	dash			
Orange rind, grated	1 tablespoon			
		71	16	60
Calories: 1 serving—115		9	2	7.5

Combine ingredients in top of double boiler. Heat until hot and bubbly.

Servings: 8
Exchange per serving: 2 vegetable, 1½ fat

Zucchini-Tomato-Onion Casserole

Ingredients	Measure	Carbohydrates (gm.)	Protein (gm.)	Fat (gm.)
Zucchini, thinly sliced	2 cups	20	8	
Tomato, thinly sliced	1	5	2	
Onion, thinly sliced	1	2.5	1	
Parmesan cheese, grated	3 tablespoons		7	5.5
		27.5	18	5.5

Calories: 1 serving—58   7   5   1

In greased 9 × 5 × 2-inch casserole, layer half of the zucchini, tomato, and onion. Sprinkle with half the cheese. Repeat. Bake uncovered at 350 degrees for 40 minutes. Cover and bake for an additional 20 minutes.

Servings: 4
Exchange per serving: 1½ vegetable, ¼ medium-fat meat

RECIPE FOR

Spectacular Salad

Ingredients	Measure	Carbohydrates (gm.)	Protein (gm.)	Fat (gm.)
Lettuce, shredded	1 head			
Hard-boiled eggs, sliced	4		28	20
Carrots, sliced	1 cup	10	4	
Frozen peas, uncooked	10 ounces	45	6	
Radishes, thinly sliced	1 cup			
Sharp cheddar cheese, shredded	1 cup		56	64
Bacon, cooked and crumbled	6 strips			30
Onion, thinly sliced	1	5	2	
		60	96	114

Calories: 1 serving—275   10   16   19

In glass bowl, layer ingredients in order listed above. Serve with favorite salad dressing. (Be sure to calculate added exchange of dressing.)

Servings: 6
Exchange per serving: 2 vegetable, 1 high-fat meat, 1 medium-fat meat, 1 fat

18

CHAPTER 4

Fruit

FRUIT EXCHANGES

One fruit exchange consists of:

Carbohydrates	10 grams
Calories	40

Fruit may be used fresh, dried, canned or frozen, cooked or raw, as long as no sugar is added.

This list shows the kinds and amounts of **fruits** to use for one fruit exchange.

Apple	1 small
Apple Juice	⅓ cup
Applesauce (unsweetened)	½ cup
Apricots, fresh	2 medium
Apricots, dried	4 halves
Banana	½ small
Berries	
Blackberries	½ cup
Blueberries	½ cup
Raspberries	½ cup
Strawberries	¾ cup
Cherries	10 large
Cider	⅓ cup
Dates	2
Figs, fresh	1
Figs, dried	1
Grapefruit	½
Grapefruit Juice	½ cup
Grapes	12
Grape Juice	¼ cup
Mango	½ small

Melon
Cantaloupe	¼ small
Honeydew	⅛ medium
Watermelon	1 cup

Nectarine	1 small
Orange	1 small
Orange Juice	½ cup
Papaya	¾ cup
Peach	1 medium
Pear	1 small
Persimmon, native	1 medium
Pineapple	½ cup
Pineapple Juice	⅓ cup
Plums	2 medium
Prunes	2 medium
Prune Juice	¼ cup
Raisins	2 tablespoons
Tangerine	1 medium

Cranberries may be used as desired if no sugar is added.

Many dessert recipes provide fruit exchanges. If you will refer to Chapter 16, you will find the following recipes can be figured in your diet as fruit exchanges:

Apple torte
Graham cracker crust
Rice crispy cereal crust
Cool-la-la lime pie filling
Cherry-cream pie filling
Fruit whip
Hawaiian dessert
Strawberry whip
Eclairs
Baked Alaska
Parfait royale

Brand-name fruit products and their exchanges are listed in an appendix at the back of the book.

Gelatin and Fruit Salad

Ingredients	Measure	Car- bohy- drates (gm.)	Pro- tein (gm.)	Fat (gm.)
Dietetic gelatin	1 envelope			
Water	1 cup			
Fruit	2 exchanges	20		
Lettuce	2 leaves			
		20		

Calories: 1 serving—40   10

Prepare gelatin according to package directions. Pour into 2 individual ring molds and chill until firm. Unmold onto lettuce and fill with 1 fruit exchange each: ½ diced banana; ½ chopped apple, sprinkled with cinnamon; ½ cup cubed pineapple.

Serving: 2
Exchange per serving: 1 fruit

Jello Mold

Ingredients	Measure	Car-bohy-drates (gm.)	Pro-tein (gm.)	Fat (gm.)
Fruit cocktail, drained (reserve juice)	2 cups	74	1.2	1.2
Cream cheese	3 ounces			30
Artificial sweetener =	3 tablespoons sugar			
Dietetic lime gelatin	3 ounces			
		74	1.2	31.2

Calories: 1 serving—97

12	.2	5

Mix jello and artificial sweetener together. Add cream cheese and dissolve in 1 cup boiling water. Add water to reserved juice to make ¾ cup. Add to mixture. Fold in fruit when mixture is partially set.

Servings: 6
Exchange per serving: 1 fruit, 1 fat

Pear Jello Mold

Ingredients	Measure	Carbohydrates (gm.)	Protein (gm.)	Fat (gm.)
Canned pear halves, drained (reserve ½ cup juice)	8	72.4	.8	.4
Dietetic lime gelatin	3 ounce package			
Cream cheese	8 ounces			80
Cool Whip	8 ounces	56		56
		128.3	.8	136.3
Calories: 1 serving—218		16	.1	17

Add ½ cup water to ½ cup pear juice and warm slightly. Add gelatin. Beat cream cheese with pears and add gelatin mixture. Fold in Cool Whip. Chill.

Servings: 8
Exchange per serving: 1 fruit, ½ bread, 3½ fat

CHAPTER 5

Bread Exchanges and Recipes

BREAD EXCHANGES

One bread exchange consists of:

Carbohydrates	15	grams
Protein	2	grams
Calories	70	

Starchy vegetables are included in this list, because they contain the same amount of carbohydrates and protein as one slice of bread.

This list shows the kinds and amounts of **breads, cereals, starchy vegetables** and prepared foods to use for one bread exchange. Those which appear in **bold type** are **low-fat.**

Bread

White (including French and Italian)	1 slice
Whole wheat	1 slice
Rye or pumpernickel	1 slice
Raisin	1 slice
Bagel, small	½
English muffin, small	½
Plain roll, bread	1
Frankfurter roll	½
Hamburger bun	½
Dried bread crumbs	3 tablespoons
Tortilla, 6″	1

24

Cereal
Bran flakes	½ cup
Other ready-to-eat unsweetened cereal	¾ cup
Puffed cereal (unfrosted)	1 cup
Cereal (cooked)	½ cup
Grits (cooked)	½ cup
Rice or barley (cooked)	½ cup
Pasta (cooked), spaghetti, noodles, macaroni	½ cup
Popcorn (popped, no fat added)	3 cups
Cornmeal (dry)	2 tablespoons
Flour	2½ tablespoons
Wheat germ	¼ cup

Crackers
Arrowroot	3
Graham, 2½" sq.	2
Matzoth, 4" × 6"	½
Oyster	20
Pretzels, 3⅛" long × ⅛" dia.	25
Rye wafers, 2" × 3½"	3
Saltines	6
Soda, 2½" sq.	4

Dried beans, peas and lentils
Beans, peas, lentils (dried and cooked)	½ cup
Baked beans, no pork (canned)	¼ cup

Starchy Vegetables
Corn	⅓ cup
Corn on cob	1 small
Lima beans	½ cup
Parsnips	⅔ cup
Peas, green (canned or frozen)	½ cup
Potato, white	1 small
Potato (mashed)	½ cup

Pumpkin	¾ cup
Winter squash, acorn or butternut	½ cup
Yam or sweet potato	¼ cup

Prepared Foods
  Biscuit 2" dia.   1
    (omit 1 fat exchange)
  Corn bread, 2" × 2" × 1"   1
    (omit 1 fat exchange)
  Corn muffin, 2" dia.   1
    (omit 1 fat exchange)
  Crackers, round butter type   5
    (omit 1 fat exchange)
  Muffin, plain small   1
    (omit 1 fat exchange)
  Potatoes, French fried, length
    2" to 3½"   8
    (omit 1 fat exchange)
  Potato or corn chips   15
    (omit 2 fat exchanges)
  Pancake, 5" × ½"   1
    (omit 1 fat exchange)
  Waffle, 5" × ½"   1
    (omit 1 fat exchange)

Brand-name bread products and their exchanges are listed in an appendix at the back of the book.

Absolutely Delicious Blueberry Muffins

Ingredients	Measure	Carbohydrates (gm.)	Protein (gm.)	Fat (gm.)
Bisquick	2 cups	152	19	29
Sour cream	1 cup			40
Egg	1		7	5
Fresh blueberries	1 cup	20		
Artificial sweetener =	6 tablespoons sugar			
Lemon peel, grated	2 teaspoons			
		172	26	74

Calories: 1 serving—118   14   2   6

Preheat oven to 425 degrees. Combine Bisquick, ¼ cup artificial sweetener. Make a well in center of mixture and add sour cream and egg, all at once. Beat with fork until well combined. Gently fold in blueberries. Put ¼ cup batter in each muffin cup. In small bowl combine lemon peel and 2 tablespoons artificial sweetener. Sprinkle over batter in each cup. Bake 20 to 25 minutes or until golden brown. Serve hot.

Servings: 12 muffins
Exchange per serving: 1 bread, 1 fat

Corn Fritters

Ingredients	Measure	Carbohydrates (gm.)	Protein (gm.)	Fat (gm.)
Frozen corn, cooked as directed	2 cups	90	12	
Flour	1 cup	96	12.8	
Baking powder	1 teaspoon			
Salt	½ teaspoon			
Pepper	¼ teaspoon			
Eggs, separated	2		14	10
Milk, skim	½ cup	6	4	
Oil for frying				
		192	42.8	10
Calories: 1 serving—84		10.6	2.3	.5

Sift flour, baking powder, salt and pepper. Beat egg whites until they form soft peaks. Beat egg yolks well; stir in corn and milk and flour mixture until blended; fold in egg whites.

Pour oil to depth of ½ inch and heat to medium. Drop rounded teaspoon of batter in oil and cook, turning once, 2 to 3 minutes, or until golden. Drain on paper towel.

Servings: 18
Exchange per serving: ¾ bread

Pineapple Fritters

Ingredients	Measure		Carbohydrates (gm.)	Protein (gm.)	Fat (gm.)
Flour, sifted	1	cup	96	12.8	.9
Artificial sweetener	2	tablespoons sugar			
	=				
Baking powder	2	teaspoons			
Salt	¼	teaspoon			
Egg	1			7	5
Milk, skim	⅔	cup	8	6	
Margarine	2	tablespoons			30
Pineapple, slices drained	10				
	1	20-ounce can	100		
			204	25.8	35
Calories: 1 serving—123			20	2.5	4

Sift flour, artificial sweetener, baking powder, and salt together. Mix egg, milk, and margarine together and stir into dry ingredients. Blend until smooth. Dip pineapple in batter, one at a time, and fry in hot fat (375 degrees) for 3 minutes, turning once. Drain on a paper towel and serve hot.

Servings: 10 fritters
Exchange per serving: 1 fruit, ¾ bread, 1 fat

Noodle Pudding

Ingredients	Measure	Carbohydrates (gm.)	Protein (gm.)	Fat (gm.)
Wide noodles, cooked and drained	10 ounces	150	20	
Eggs, beaten	3		21	15
Artificial sweetener	= ¾ cup sugar			
Pineapple, crushed	1 8-ounce can	40		
Apples, peeled and grated	5	50		
Maraschino cherries	8	40		
Cinnamon	to taste			
Oil	4 tablespoons			60
		280	41	75
Calories: 1 serving—123		17	2.5	4.5

Heat 1 tablespoon oil in pan. Combine remaining ingredients and pour into pan. Let set for 24 hours. Bake 1 hour at 350 degrees.

Servings: 16

Exchange per serving: 1 bread, 1 fat

Popovers

Ingredients	Measure	Carbohydrates (gm.)	Protein (gm.)	Fat (gm.)
Eggs	2		14	10
Milk, skim	1 cup	12	8	
Flour	1 cup	96	12.8	
Salt	¼ teaspoon			
Margarine, melted	1 tablespoon			15
		108	35	25
Calories: 1 serving—66		9	3	2

Beat eggs and add milk as you continue to beat. Sift flour and salt together and add to egg and milk mixture as you continue to beat. Add melted margarine. Pour batter into 12 small popover cups. Bake at 425 degrees for 35 minutes.

Servings: 12
Exchange per serving: ¾ bread, ⅓ fat

Quick Blender Popovers

Ingredients	Measure	Car-bohy-drates (gm.)	Pro-tein (gm.)	Fat (gm.)
Milk, skim	1 cup	12	8	
Eggs	2		14	10
Flour, sifted	1 cup	96	12.8	
Salt	¼ teaspoon			
		108	34.8	10
Calories: 1 serving—55		9	3	.8

Put all ingredients in blender. Cover and blend on high speed for 15 seconds. Pour into greased muffin pans and bake at 425 degrees for 40 minutes.

Servings: 12
Exchange per serving: ¾ bread

Yorkshire Pudding

Ingredients	Measure	Car-bohy-drates (gm.)	Pro-tein (gm.)	Fat (gm.)
Eggs	2		14	10
Milk, skim	1 cup	12	8	
Flour	1 cup	96	12.8	
Salt	½ teaspoon			
Roast beef drippings	2 tablespoons			30
		108	34.8	40
Calories: 1 serving—97		9	4	5

As soon as roast beef has been removed from the oven, increase oven temperature to 425 degrees. In a medium bowl beat eggs, milk, flour, and salt to make a smooth batter. Pour drippings into a 10-inch pie plate (or six individual custard cups); tilt to coat bottom and side of pie plate. Pour in batter. Bake 25 minutes or until the pudding is deep golden brown. Serve immediately with the roast beef.

Servings: 8
Exchange per serving: 2 vegetable, 1 fat

RECIPE FOR

Muffins

Ingredients	Measure	Car-bohy-drates (gm.)	Pro-tein (gm.)	Fat (gm.)
Flour	1½ cups	144	19.2	
Double-acting baking powder	3 teaspoons			
Salt	½ teaspoon			
Egg, slightly beaten	1		7	5
Milk, skim	¾ cup	9	6	
Vegetable oil	2 tablespoons			30
Artificial sweetener =	8 teaspoons sugar			
		153	32.2	35
Calories: 1 serving—128		19	4	4

Sift flour, baking powder, and salt together. Combine egg, milk, oil, and artificial sweetener. Add liquid mixture to dry ingredients, mixing until all dry particles are moistened. Fill well greased muffin cups two-thirds full. Bake at 400 degrees for 25 minutes.

Servings: 8
Exchange per serving: 1½ bread, 1 fat

Apple Muffins

Ingredients	Measure	Carbohy-drates (gm.)	Pro-tein (gm.)	Fat (gm.)
Flour	1⅔ cups	160	21	1.5
Artificial sweetener	16 teaspoons = sugar			
Baking powder	2½ teaspoons			
Salt	½ teaspoon			
Cinnamon	1 teaspoon			
Nutmeg	¼ teaspoon			
Egg, lightly beaten	1		7	5
Margarine, melted	¼ cup			60
Milk	⅔ cup	8	6	
Apples, minced	1 cup	20		
		188	34	65
Calories: 1 serving—119		15.6	3	5

Sift flour, artificial sweetener, baking powder, salt, and spices into mixing bowl. Combine egg, milk, and margarine; add to dry ingredients. Blend until flour is moistened. Do not overmix or batter will be lumpy. Fold in apples. Pour batter into greased muffin cups filling until two-thirds full. Bake at 400 degrees for 25 minutes.

Servings: 12
Exchange per serving: 1 bread, 1 fat

Orange Marmalade Nut Bread

Ingredients	Measure	Carbohydrates (gm.)	Protein (gm.)	Fat (gm.)
Flour	2 cups	192	25.6	
Baking powder	1½ teaspoons			
Baking soda	½ teaspoon			
Salt	¼ teaspoon			
Milk, skim	⅓ cup	4	2.6	
Egg	1		7	5
Margarine, melted	2 tablespoons			30
Artificial sweetener =	8 tablespoons sugar			
Dietetic orange marmalade	½ cup			
Walnuts, chopped	¼ cup			20
		196	35	55
Calories: 1 serving—112		16	3	4

Combine flour, baking powder, baking soda, and salt in a mixing bowl. Combine milk, egg, margarine, and artificial sweetener; add to flour mixture. Stir only until all flour is moistened. Fold in marmalade and chopped nuts, mixing as little as possible. Spoon batter into lightly greased loaf pan. Bake at 350 degrees for 1 hour. Cool before slicing.

Servings: 12
Exchange per serving: 1 bread, 1 fat

Banana Nut Bread

Ingredients	Measure	Carbohydrates (gm.)	Protein (gm.)	Fat (gm.)
Ripe bananas, mashed	3	60		
Artificial sweetener, granulated =	24 teaspoons sugar			
Eggs, well beaten	2		14	10
Flour	1¾ cups	168	22	
Baking powder	3 teaspoons			
Salt	¼ teaspoon			
Walnuts, chopped	¼ cup			20
		228	36	30
Calories: 1 serving—98		19	3	2.5

Sprinkle artificial sweetener over bananas and mix well; blend in eggs. Sift together flour, baking powder, and salt; add walnuts; blend thoroughly into banana mixture but do not overmix. Pour into loaf pan. Bake at 325 degrees for 55 minutes.

Servings: 12
Exchange per serving: 1 bread, ½ fruit, ½ fat

Stuffed Baked Potatoes

Ingredients	Measure	Car- bohy- drates (gm.)	Pro- tein (gm.)	Fat (gm.)
Baking potatoes	4	60	8	
Onion, minced	¼ cup	2.5	1	
Salt	1 teaspoon			
Pepper	⅛ teaspoon			
Margarine	1 tablespoon			15
Egg	1		7	5
Sour cream	4 tablespoons			10
		62.5	16	30
Calories: 1 serving—141		15.8	4	7.5

Bake potatoes at 400 degrees for 1 hour. Remove from oven and cut in half lengthwise. Remove pulp, reserving skins. Place pulp in mixing bowl. Add onion, salt, pepper, margarine, and egg. Beat well, until fluffy. Refill potato skins and arrange in a shallow baking dish with cut sides up. Spoon sour cream over each half. Bake 10 minutes until tops are lightly browned.

Servings: 4
Exchange per serving: 1 bread, 1½ fat

Oven Browned Potato Sticks

Ingredients	Measure	Carbohydrates (gm.)	Protein (gm.)	Fat (gm.)
Large potatoes, sliced into sticks	8	120	16	
Salad oil	½ cup			120
Salt	1 teaspoon			
		120	16	120
Calories: 1 serving—203		15	2	15

Place salad oil in a large shallow baking pan; roll potato sticks in oil to coat well, then arrange in a single layer in same pan; sprinkle with salt. Bake at 400 degrees for 1 hour, or until tender and crusty-golden.

Servings: 8
Exchange per serving: 1 bread, 3 fat

Potato Cake

Ingredients	Measure	Carbohydrates (gm.)	Protein (gm.)	Fat (gm.)
Medium potatoes, peeled	6	90	12	
Margarine	4 tablespoons			60
Salt	as desired			
Pepper	as desired			
		90	12	60
Calories: 1 serving—158		15	2	10

Slice potatoes thinly and evenly. Butter 1½-quart baking dish. Arrange layer of potatoes over bottom and sides. Dot with margarine. Sprinkle with salt and pepper. Repeat until dish is full. Cover. Bake at 400 degrees for 1 hour. Carefully turn out on warm platter.

Servings: 6
Exchange per serving: 1 bread, 2 fat

Escalloped Potatoes

Ingredients	Measure	Carbohydrates (gm.)	Protein (gm.)	Fat (gm.)
Potato, peeled	1 small	15	2	
Salt	as desired			
Pepper	as desired			
Onion, chopped	½ teaspoon			
Milk, skim	½ cup	6	4	
Margarine	1 teaspoon			5
Calories: 1 serving—153		21	6	5

Slice potato and place half the slices in bottom of individual casserole. Sprinkle lightly with salt, pepper, and chopped onion. Cover with remaining potato slices; sprinkle with salt and pepper and add milk. Dot top with margarine. Bake in moderate oven (350 degrees) about 45 minutes.

Servings: 1
Exchange per serving: 1 bread, ½ milk, 1 fat

Quick Scalloped Potatoes

Ingredients	Measure	Car-bohy-drates (gm.)	Pro-tein (gm.)	Fat (gm.)
Cheddar cheese soup	1 10½-ounce can	24.9	14.4	29.7
Milk, skim	½ cup	6	4	
Potatoes, thinly sliced	4 cups	60	8	
Onion, thinly sliced	1	7	2	
Margarine	1 tablespoon			15
Paprika	as desired			
		97.9	28.4	44.7
Calories: 1 serving—150.6		16.3	4.7	7.4

Stir soup until smooth; gradually add milk. In buttered casserole arrange alternate layers of potato, onion, and the cheese sauce. Dot top with margarine. Sprinkle with paprika. Bake, covered, at 375 degrees for 1 hour. Uncover, bake 15 minutes more.

Servings: 6
Exchange per serving: 1 bread, ½ meat, ½ fat

Crisp Baked Potato Halves

Ingredients	Measure	Carbohydrates (gm.)	Protein (gm.)	Fat (gm.)
Baking potatoes	4 medium	60	8	
Margarine	4 tablespoons			60
Salt	as desired			
Pepper	as desired			
		60	8	60
Calories: 1 serving—203		15	2	15

Scrub potatoes and cut in half lengthwise. Score cut side of each half with a fork; brush with margarine and sprinkle with salt and pepper. Place potatoes on a cookie sheet, cut sides up, and bake at 400 degrees for 40 minutes, until fork tender.

Servings: 4
Exchange per serving: 1 bread, 3 fat

Potato Salad

Ingredients	Measure	Car-bohy-drates (gm.)	Pro-tein (gm.)	Fat (gm.)
Potatoes, cooked and finely diced	6 cups (6)	90	12	
Onion, grated	1	5	2	
Chopped dill pickle	3 tablespoons			
Mayonnaise	½ cup			120
Prepared mustard	1½ teaspoons			
Salt	½ teaspoon			
Pepper	⅛ teaspoon			
		95	14	120
Calories: 1 serving—252		16.1	2.3	20

Combine all ingredients and refrigerate. You can use this recipe for macaroni salad by substituting 3 cups cooked macaroni for the potatoes.

Servings: 6
Exchange per serving: 1 bread, 4 fat

Mushroom Potato Pie

Ingredients	Measure	Car-bohy-drates (gm.)	Pro-tein (gm.)	Fat (gm.)
Potatoes, mashed	3 cups	90	12	
Mushrooms, sliced	1½ cups	15	6	
Onion, minced	¼ cup	2.5	1	
Margarine	2 tablespoons			30
Lemon juice	1 teaspoon			
Salt	as desired			
Pepper	⅛ teaspoon			
Sour cream	½ cup			20
		107.5	19	50
Calories: 1 serving—156		18	3	8

Place half the mashed potatoes in a layer in a buttered 9-inch pie pan. Sauté mushrooms and onion in hot margarine. Stir in lemon juice, salt, and pepper. Top potatoes with mushrooms and sour cream. Cover with remaining potatoes. Bake at 350 degrees about 35 minutes.

Servings: 6
Exchange per serving: 1 bread, ½ vegetable, 1½ fat

Potato and Onion in Foil

Ingredients	Measure	Car-bohy-drates (gm.)	Pro-tein (gm.)	Fat (gm.)
Baking potato	1 medium	15	2	
Onion, thinly sliced	1 medium	5	2	
Margarine	2 teaspoons			10
Salt	½ teaspoon			
Paprika	as desired			
Calories: 1 serving—186		20	4	10

Place potato, cut into ¼-inch slices, on piece of aluminum foil. Insert an onion slice between each 2 potato slices. Spread potato with margarine, salt, and paprika. Bring foil together and fold over to seal. Place on baking sheet. Bake at 425 degrees for 45 minutes, or until tender.

Servings: 1
Exchange per serving: 1 bread, 1 vegetable, 2 fat

Bread Stuffing

Ingredients	Measure	Carbohydrates (gm.)	Protein (gm.)	Fat (gm.)
Bread	1 slice	15	2	
Onion, chopped	½ teaspoon			
Salt	pinch			
Pepper	a few grains			
Poultry seasoning	⅛ teaspoon			
Margarine, melted	1 teaspoon			5
Water	to moisten			
Calories: 1 serving—113		15	2	5

Cut bread into cubes. Add onion, seasonings, and margarine; mix well. Add water to moisten.

Servings: 1
Exchange per serving: 1 bread, 1 fat

Party Mix

Ingredients	Measure	Carbohydrates (gm.)	Protein (gm.)	Fat (gm.)
Margarine	8 tablespoons			120
Worcestershire sauce	4½ teaspoons			
Seasoned salt	1¼ teaspoons			
Rice Chex	2 cups	44	2.8	
Corn Chex	2 cups	50	4	
Wheat Chex	2 cups	46	6	
Peanuts	1 cup	66	104	199
		206	116.8	319
Calories: 1 serving—297		15	8	23

Preheat oven to 250 degrees. Melt margarine in shallow pan. Stir in Worcestershire sauce and seasoned salt. Add remaining ingredients and stir until coated. Heat in oven 45 minutes, stirring every 15 minutes. Cool. Can store in airtight container.

Servings: 14 half-cup servings
Exchange per serving: 1 bread, 1 high-fat meat, 3 fat

Apple Nut Bread

Ingredients	Measure	Car-bohy-drates (gm.)	Pro-tein (gm.)	Fat (gm.)
Margarine	¼ cup			60
Brown sugar	1 cup	204		
Eggs	2		14	10
All purpose flour, unsifted	3 cups	288	38	
Baking soda	1½ teaspoons			
Baking powder	1 teaspoon			
Salt	1 teaspoon			
Lemon rind, grated	½ teaspoon			
Nuts, chopped	¾ cup			60
Cinnamon	1 teaspoon			
Nutmeg	¼ teaspoon			
Apple, pared and grated	2 small	20		
Buttermilk	¾ cup	9	6	8
		521	58	138
Calories: 1 serving—288		43	2	12

In medium bowl cream margarine and sugar. Beat in eggs. Mix flour, soda, baking powder, salt, lemon rind, nuts, cinnamon, nutmeg, and grated apple. Blend into creamed mixture alternately with buttermilk. Turn into greased and floured 9 × 5 × 3-inch loaf pan and bake 1 hour at 350 degrees. Cool for 10 minutes, remove from pan, and cool on wire rack.

Servings: 12
Exchange per serving: 1 fruit, 2 bread, 2½ fat

RECIPE FOR

Supreme Spinach

Ingredients	Measure	Carbohydrates (gm.)	Protein (gm.)	Fat (gm.)
Bisquick baking mix	1 cup	76	9.5	14.5
Milk, skim	¼ cup	3	2	
Eggs	2		14	10
Onion, finely chopped	¼ cup	2.5	1	
Chopped spinach, thawed and drained	10 ounces	7.2	7.5	.7
Parmesan cheese, grated	9 tablespoons		21	16.5
Monterey Jack cheese, cubed	4 ounces		28	22
Creamed cottage cheese	12 ounces		21	16.5
Salt	½ teaspoon			
Garlic, crushed	2 cloves			
Eggs	2		14	10
		88.7	118	90.1

Calories: 1 serving—205   11   15   11

Heat oven to 375 degrees. Grease 12×7½×2-inch baking dish. Mix Bisquick, milk, 2 eggs, and onion; beat vigorously. Spread in dish. Mix remaining ingredients and spoon evenly over batter in dish. Bake 30 minutes or until set. Let stand 5 minutes before cutting.

Servings: 8
Exchange per serving: ⅔ bread, 2 medium-fat meat

Potato Squares

Ingredients	Measure	Car-bohy-drates (gm.)	Pro-tein (gm.)	Fat (gm.)
Mashed potatoes	3 cups	90	12	
Flour	2 tablespoons	12	1.6	
Salt	1½ teaspoons			
Pepper	¼ teaspoon			
Sour cream	½ cup			20
Chives, chopped	2 tablespoons			
Egg, slightly beaten	1		7	5.5
Swiss cheese, shredded	½ cup		28	12
Bacon, crisp and crumbled	4 slices			20
		162	48.5	57.5

Calories: 1 serving—187   17   8   10

Mix potatoes, flour, salt, and pepper. Spoon into greased 9 × 9 × 2-inch baking dish. Mix sour cream, chives, and egg. Spread over potato mixture. Sprinkle with cheese and bacon. Bake at 350 degrees 25 to 30 minutes or until set. Cut in squares.

Servings: 6
Exchange per serving: 1 bread, 1 medium-fat meat, 1 fat

CHAPTER 6

Meat Exchanges and Recipes

MEAT EXCHANGES

One low-fat meat exchange consists of:

Protein	7 grams
Fat	3 grams
Calories	55

One medium-fat meat exchange consists of:

Protein	7 grams
Fat	5.5 grams
Calories	77.5

One high-fat meat exchange consists of:

Protein	7 grams
Fat	8 grams
Calories	100

This list shows the kinds and amounts of **lean meat** and other protein-rich foods to use for one low-fat meat exchange.

Beef:	Baby beef (very lean), chipped beef, chuck, flank steak, Tenderloin, plate ribs, plate skirt steak, round (bottom, top), all cuts rump, spare ribs, tripe	1 ounce
Lamb:	Leg, rib, sirloin, loin (roast and chops), shank, shoulder	1 ounce
Pork:	Leg (whole rump, center shank), ham, smoked (center slices)	1 ounce
Veal:	Leg, loin, rib, shank, shoulder, cutlets	1 ounce
Poultry:	Meat without skin of chicken, turkey, Cornish hen, Guinea hen, pheasant	1 ounce

Fish:	Any fresh or frozen	1 ounce
	Canned salmon, tuna, mackerel, crab and lobster,	¼ cup
	Clams, oysters, scallops, shrimp,	5 or 1 ounce
	Sardines, drained	3
Cheeses containing less than 5% butterfat		1 ounce
Cottage cheese, dry and 2% butterfat		¼ cup
Dried beans and peas (omit 1 bread exchange)		½ cup

This list shows the kinds and amounts of medium-fat meat and other protein-rich foods to use for one medium-fat meat exchange.

Beef:	Ground (15% fat), corned beef (canned), rib eye, round (ground commercial)	1 ounce
Pork:	Loin (all cuts tenderloin), shoulder arm (picnic), shoulder blade, Boston butt, Canadian bacon, boiled ham	1 ounce
Liver, heart, kidney and sweetbreads (these are high in cholesterol)		1 ounce
Cottage cheese, creamed		¼ cup
Cheese:	mozzarella, ricotta, farmer's cheese, neufchatel,	1 ounce
	Parmesan	3 teaspoons
Egg (high in cholesterol)		1
Peanut butter (omit 2 additional fat exchanges)		2 teaspoons

This list shows the kinds and amounts of high-fat meat and other protein-rich foods to use for one high-fat meat exchange.

Beef:	Brisket, corned beef (brisket), ground beef (more than 20% fat), hamburger (commercial), chuck (ground commercial), roasts (rib), steaks (club and rib)	1 ounce

53

Lamb:	Breast	1 ounce
Pork:	Spare ribs, loin (back ribs), pork (ground), country style ham, deviled ham	1 ounce
Veal:	Breast	1 ounce
Poultry:	Capon, duck (domestic), goose	1 ounce
Cheese:	Cheddar types	1 ounce
Cold cuts		4½" × ⅛" slice
Frankfurter		1 small

BROILING

Meat broiled can be calculated as 1 meat exchange per ounce of cooked meat.

Suitable Cuts for Broiling

Beef
Club steak
Top quality chuck steak
Patties
Porterhouse steak
Tenderloin
Top quality top round
T-bone steak
Rib steak
Sirloin steak

Lamb
Loin chops
Rib chops
Shoulder chops
Patties
Steak

Pork
Bacon
Ham
Loin chops
Rib chops
Shoulder chops

Veal
Loin chops

PAN BROILING

Meat pan broiled (in Teflon-type coated pans to eliminate the use of fat) can be calculated as 1 meat exchange per ounce of cooked meat.

Suitable Cuts for Pan Broiling

Bacon
Beef or lamb patties
Cubed steak
Ham
Lamb chops
Sausage
Steaks, less than 1-inch thick

ROASTING

Meat roasted can be calculated as 1 meat exchange per ounce of cooked meat.

Suitable Cuts for Roasting

Beef—300°
Choice quality chuck ribs
Rolled ribs
Rump
Standing ribs
Tenderloin
Choice quality top round

Lamb—300°
Leg
Loin
Ribs
Shoulder

Pork—350°
Boston butt
Crown roast
Fresh or smoked ham
Loin
Picnic shoulder

Veal—300°
Leg
Loin
Shoulder

Roast in slow oven, on rack, without adding water or other liquid. Roast 20 to 30 minutes per pound for beef; 25 to 40 minutes per pound for veal; 25 to 45 minutes per pound for pork; 30 to 40 minutes per pound for lamb.

Internal Temperatures of Roasts When Done

Cut	Rare	Medium	Well done
Beef	140°	160°	170°
Lamb		175°	180°
Pork			185°
Veal			170°
Ham			170°

Brand-name meat products and their exchanges are listed in an appendix at the back of the book.

Liver and Onion

Ingredients	Measure	Carbohy-drates (gm.)	Pro-tein (gm.)	Fat (gm.)
Margarine	6 tablespoons			90
Onion, frozen, chopped	1½ cups	15	6	
Flour	¼ cup	24	3.2	
Salt	2 teaspoons			
Paprika	2 teaspoons			
Beef liver, sliced	2 pounds		168	132
		39	177.2	222

Calories: 1 serving—477   6.5   29.5   37

Combine 4 tablespoons margarine and onions in frying pan; heat slowly until margarine melts; cover pan and cook slowly 5 minutes. Uncover and cook, stirring several times, 10 minutes or until golden. Mix flour, salt, and paprika in pie plate and coat liver pieces. Sauté in remaining margarine in frying pan 4 minutes on each side, or until done as you like it. Serve on serving platter and surround with onions.

Servings: 6
Exchange per serving: 4 medium-fat meat, ½ bread, 3 fat

Baked Tongue

Ingredients	Measure	Car- bohy- drates (gm.)	Pro- tein (gm.)	Fat (gm.)
Tongue, pickled or smoked				
Water	½ cup			

Place tongue in casserole; add water; cover and bake at 350 degrees for 50 minutes per pound.

Exchange per serving: 1 high-fat meat exchange per ounce in serving.

RECIPE FOR

Danish Salad Mold

Ingredients	Measure	Car- bohy- drates (gm.)	Pro- tein (gm.)	Fat (gm.)
Potatoes, cooked and finely diced	6 cups (6)	90	12	
Onion, grated	1	5	2	
Chopped dill pickle	3 tablespoons			
Mayonnaise	½ cup			120
Prepared mustard	1½ teaspoons			
Salt	½ teaspoon			
Pepper	⅛ teaspoon			
Beef tongue, cooked	12 1-ounce slices		84	35
Lettuce				
		95	98	196
Calories: 1 serving—361.8		16	16	33

Combine potatoes, onion, pickle, mayonnaise, and seasonings; mix well. Line lightly oiled 6-cup mixing bowl with tongue slices, slightly overlapping, with rounded ends toward bottom of bowl; fill with potato salad mixture, pressing down lightly all over to fill bowl. Chill 1 hour. When ready to serve loosen meat around edge of bowl; turn bowl upside down on serving plate and lift off. Garnish with lettuce.

Servings: 6
Exchange per serving: 2 high-fat meat, 1 bread, 3 fat

59

Combination Salad

Ingredients	Measure	Carbohydrates (gm.)	Protein (gm.)	Fat (gm.)
American cheese, in strips	1 ounce		7	3
Cold cuts, in strips	2 ounces		14	16
Egg, hard boiled	1		7	2.5
Lettuce, shredded	¼ small head			
Onion, sliced	1 small	5	2	
Tomato, quartered	1	5	2	
Raw cauliflowerets, asparagus spears, peas, etc., cooked	as desired			
Vinegar	2 tablespoons			
Salad oil	2 teaspoons			10
Calories: 1 serving—447		10	32	31

Combine first 7 ingredients; season as desired. Pour vinegar over; pour oil over and toss to coat well.

Servings: 1
Exchange per serving: 4 high-fat meat, 2 vegetable

Flank Steak

Ingredients	Measure	Carbohydrates (gm.)	Protein (gm.)	Fat (gm.)
Flank steak	1 pound		84	36
Vegetable oil	1 cup			
Vinegar	½ cup			
Salt	1 teaspoon			
Pepper	¼ teaspoon			
Dry mustard	2 teaspoons			
Worcestershire sauce	2 teaspoons			
Cayenne	a dash			
Tabasco sauce	a few drops			

Calories: 1 serving—165

Place steak in pan. Combine remaining ingredients and pour over steak. Let stand at least 3 hours. Remove from marinade and broil 5 minutes on each side 2 inches from fire. Carve diagonally across grain into thin slices. (Discard marinade.)

Servings: 4
Exchange per serving: 3 low-fat meat

Chopped Chicken Livers

Ingredients	Measure	Carbohydrates (gm.)	Protein (gm.)	Fat (gm.)
Oil	2 tablespoons			30
Onions, sliced	2 small	10	4	
Chicken livers	½ pound		42	33
Water	2 tablespoons			
Eggs, hard-boiled, chopped	2		14	5
Salt	½ teaspoon			
Pepper	a few grains			
Chicken broth	3 tablespoons			
		10	60	68
Calories: 1 2-ounce serving—182		20	12	14

Heat oil in skillet; add onion and cook until tender, stirring occasionally. Add livers and cook until lightly browned. Add water; cover and cook slowly 10 minutes. Cool and chop livers finely. Mix livers, egg, salt, and pepper. Stir in broth to moisten.

Servings: 5
Exchange per serving: ½ vegetable, 1½ medium-fat meat, 1 fat

CHAPTER 7

Beef Recipes

Beef Stew With Dumplings

Ingredients	Measure		Carbohydrates (gm.)	Protein (gm.)	Fat (gm.)
Boneless beef chuck, cut into 1-inch cubes	1	pound		84	36
Hot water	2	cups			
Lemon juice	½	teaspoon			
Worcestershire sauce	½	teaspoon			
Garlic, minced	½	clove			
Onion, sliced	½				
Bay leaf, crumbled	1	small			
Salt	1	teaspoon			
Pepper	¼	teaspoon			
Artificial sweetener =	½	teaspoon sugar			
Carrots, halved	3		25	10	
Onions	4	small	15	6	
Potatoes, quartered	2		30	4	
Dumplings (recipe page 66)			80.5	12.5	50.5
			150.5	116.5	50.5
Calories: 1 serving—385			38	29	13

Brown meat thoroughly on all sides (about 30 minutes) in heavy pan. Add all ingredients except vegetables. Cover tightly. Cook 2 hours. Add vegetables, cook 10 minutes. Add dumplings; finish cooking with dumplings.

Servings: 4
Exchange per serving: 2 bread, 4 low-fat meat, 1 vegetable

Dumplings

Ingredients	Measure	Carbohydrates (gm.)	Protein (gm.)	Fat (gm.)
Bisquick	1 cup	76	9.5	14.5
Milk, skim	6 tablespoons	4.5	3	
		80.5	12.5	14.5
Calories: 1 serving—125.2		20.1	3.1	3.6

Mix milk with Bisquick. Spoon batter lightly onto bubbling stew. Cook 10 minutes uncovered and 10 minutes covered. Remove. Top stew with dumplings on warm plates.

Servings: 4
Exchange per serving: 1½ bread, ½ fat

Barbecued Chuck Roast

Ingredients	Measure	Car-bohy-drates (gm.)	Pro-tein (gm.)	Fat (gm.)
Chuck roast, boneless	2 pounds, 2-inches thick		168	72
Monosodium glutamate	1 teaspoon			
Wine vinegar	⅓ cup			
Catsup	¼ cup	19.6	1.6	
Salad oil	2 tablespoons			30
Soy sauce	2 tablespoons			
Worcestershire sauce	1 tablespoon			
Garlic salt	1 teaspoon			
Prepared mustard	1 teaspoon			
Pepper	¼ teaspoon			
		19.6	169.6	102
Calories: 1 serving—209		2.4	21.2	13

Wipe meat, sprinkle with monosodium glutamate, and place in shallow baking dish. Combine all remaining ingredients; mix well; pour over meat and refrigerate, covered, 2 to 3 hours, turning meat several times. Take meat out of marinade, sprinkle with monosodium glutamate, and broil 6 inches from heat for 50 minutes, turning every 10 minutes and brushing with marinade.

Servings: 8
Exchange per serving: 3 low-fat meat, 1 fat

Brisket Dinner

Ingredients	Measure	Carbohydrates (gm.)	Protein (gm.)	Fat (gm.)
Beef brisket, boneless	2 pounds		168	192
Water	1 cup			
Beef bouillon cubes	2			
Garlic, minced	1 clove			
Bay leaf	1			
Onion, peeled	1			
Cloves, whole	8			
Onions, peeled	4	20	8	
Carrots, in 2-inch cubes	6	50	20	
Salt	2 teaspoons			
Pepper	¼ teaspoon			
Mushrooms, fresh	6 large			
Flour	2½ tablespoons	15	2	
		85	198	192
Calories: 1 serving—360		11.1	25	24

Brown beef; stir in water, bouillon cubes, garlic, and bay leaf. Stud onion with cloves; drop into pan; cover. Simmer 1½ hours, turning meat once. Place onions and carrots in liquid around meat, sprinkle with salt and pepper, and cover again. Simmer 45 minutes. Add mushrooms and simmer 15 minutes. Remove meat to heated platter, place vegetables around edge, discarding bay leaf and onion with cloves; keep hot while making gravy.

Pour liquid into 4-cup measure; let stand about a minute. Skim off fat and measure 3 tablespoons back into pan. Add water, if needed, to make 3 cups. Blend flour into fat in pan; cook, stirring constantly, just until bubbly. Stir in the 3 cups liquid; continue cooking, stirring constantly, until gravy thickens and boils one minute. Serve slices of meat with gravy.

Servings: 8
Exchange per serving: 2 vegetable, 3 high-fat meat

RECIPE FOR

Lipton Pot Roast in Onion Sauce

Ingredients	Measure	Carbohydrates (gm.)	Protein (gm.)	Fat (gm.)
Boneless pot roast of beef	3 pounds		252	198
Water	2 cups			
Lipton onion soup mix	1 envelope	30	4	

Brown meat well. Add water and soup mix. Simmer, covered, 3 hours, or until meat is tender, turning occasionally.

Exchange per serving: 1 medium-fat meat exchange per ounce serving.

70

Man-Style Meat and Potatoes

Ingredients	Measure	Carbohy-drates (gm.)	Pro-tein (gm.)	Fat (gm.)
Beef, cooked, cut into strips	1½ cups		84	66
Onion, thinly sliced	1	5	2	
Margarine	2 tablespoons			30
Cream of celery soup	1 10½-ounce can	19.2	4.2	11.7
Milk, skim	⅓ cup	4	2.6	
Cheddar cheese, shredded	1 cup		56	64
Pepper	dash			
Potatoes, cooked and sliced	3 cups	90	12	
Paprika	dash			
		118.2	160.8	168.4
Calories: 1 serving—667		30	40	42

In sauce pan, brown beef and cook onion in margarine until onion is tender. Blend in soup, milk, ¾ cup cheese, and pepper. In a 1½-quart casserole arrange alternating layers of potatoes, meat, onion, and sauce. Sprinkle with remaining cheese and paprika. Bake uncovered at 375 degrees for 30 minutes.

Servings: 4
Exchange per serving: 2 bread, 3 medium-fat meat, 2 high-fat meat, 2 fat

Steak-Potato Casserole

Ingredients	Measure	Carbohydrates (gm.)	Protein (gm.)	Fat (gm.)
Round steak	1 pound		84	36
Flour	2½ tablespoons	15	2	
Margarine	3 tablespoons			45
Potatoes, peeled and sliced	4	45	6	
Onion, chopped	1	5	2	
Parsley, chopped	a few sprigs			
Salt	½ teaspoon			
Pepper	⅛ teaspoon			
Tomato sauce	16 ounces	56	16	
		121	110	81
Calories: 1 serving—412		30	28	20

Cut meat into 4 serving pieces and dredge in flour. Brown in margarine on both sides in Dutch oven. Add potatoes and next four ingredients. Pour tomato sauce over top. Cover and bake in moderate oven (350 degrees) about 1½ hours.

Servings: 4
Exchange per serving: 2 low-fat meat, 2 bread, 2 fat

Spanish Rice—Using Leftover Beef

Ingredients	Measure	Car-bohy-drates (gm.)	Pro-tein (gm.)	Fat (gm.)
Green pepper, chopped	½ cup	5	2	
Onion, chopped	½ cup	5	2	
Rice, cooked	1½ cups	45	6	
Oil	¼ cup			60
Beef broth	1 cup			
Tomato sauce	16 ounces	56	16	
Salt	½ teaspoon			
Pepper	⅛ teaspoon			
Beef, cooked and diced	1½ cups		84	66
		111	110	126
Calories: 1 serving—512		28	28	32

Saute green pepper, onion and rice in oil, stirring until lightly brown. Add broth, tomato sauce, salt, pepper and beef. Bring to boil, reduce heat, and simmer uncovered 5 minutes.

Servings: 4
Exchange per serving: 3 medium-fat meat, 2½ vegetable, 1 bread, 3 fat

Savory Brisket

Ingredients	Measure	Carbohydrates (gm.)	Protein (gm.)	Fat (gm.)
Brisket	4 pounds		336	384
Onion soup mix	1 envelope	30	4	
Apricot nectar	46 ounces	165.6	3.4	1.15
		195.6	343.4	385
Calories: 1 serving—468		16	29	32

Salt, pepper, and flour brisket. Brown, without adding additional fat, in Teflon-type pan. Move to baking pan, add soup mix and nectar. Cover and bake at 350 degrees for 2½ hours.

Can cool, slice, return to gravy, and freeze, if desired.

Servings: 12
Exchange per serving: 1½ fruit, 4 high-fat meat

CHAPTER 8

Lamb and Veal Recipes

Shoulder Lamb Chops, Shaslik Style

Ingredients	Measure	Carbohydrates (gm.)	Protein (gm.)	Fat (gm.)
Shoulder lamb chops	6 5-ounce chops, excluding bone		158	68
Vegetable oil	½ cup			
Red wine vinegar	2 tablespoons			
Lemon juice	2 tablespoons			
Garlic salt	1 teaspoon			
Pepper	¼ teaspoon			
Oregano	½ teaspoon			
Bay leaf, crumpled	½			

Calories: 1 serving—292

Place chops in shallow pan. Mix remaining ingredients, pour over chops, cover. Marinate at least 24 hours, turning occasionally. Remove chops from marinade and broil 3 inches from fire about 12 minutes. (Discard marinade.)

Servings: 6
Exchange per serving: 4 low-fat meat

Glazed Lamb Chops with Onions

Ingredients	Measure	Carbohydrates (gm.)	Protein (gm.)	Fat (gm.)
Shoulder lamb chops	8 5-ounce chops excluding bone		210	90
Small white onions, drained	1 16-ounce can	28	8	
Frozen orange juice concentrate	1 6-ounce can	60		
Salt	as desired			
Pepper	as desired			
		88	318	90
Calories: 1 serving—251		11	27	11

Season chops with salt and pepper and lightly brown on both sides in skillet. Arrange chops and onions in shallow roasting pan. Heat orange juice concentrate with pan drippings; pour over chops. Cover. Bake at 350 degrees for 30 minutes. Uncover; bake 15 minutes more, or until tender, basting frequently.

Servings: 8
Exchange per serving: 4 low-fat meat, 1 fruit

Veal Parmigiana

Ingredients	Measure	Car-bohy-drates (gm.)	Pro-tein (gm.)	Fat (gm.)
Veal steak, very thin	1 pound		84	36
Onion, minced	1	5	2	
Olive oil	3 tablespoons			45
Tomatoes	1 19-ounce can	20	8	
Garlic salt	1¼ teaspoons			
Pepper	¼ teaspoon			
Tomato sauce	1 8-ounce can	28	8	
Oregano	dash			
Dry bread crumbs	¼ cup	20	3	
Parmesan cheese, grated	2 ounces		18	14
Egg, beaten	1		7	5
Mozzarella cheese	½ pound		56	44
		73	186	144
Calories: 1 serving—584		18	47	35

Cut veal in serving-size pieces. Cook onion in 1 tablespoon olive oil 5 minutes. Add tomatoes, broken with fork; add garlic salt and pepper. Simmer, uncovered, 10 minutes. Add tomato sauce and oregano. Simmer 20 minutes longer. Mix bread crumbs and ¼ cup grated cheese. Dip veal in egg, then in crumbs. Brown in 2 tablespoons oil in skillet. Put in shallow baking dish. Pour about ⅔ sauce over veal; top with mozzarella, then rest of sauce. Sprinkle with grated cheese. Bake at 375 degrees for 30 minutes.

Servings: 4
Exchange per serving: 1 vegetable, 1 bread, 3 low-fat meat, 3 medium-fat meat, 1 fat

Shish Kabob

Ingredients	Measure	Car-bohy-drates (gm.)	Pro-tein (gm.)	Fat (gm.)
Leg of lamb, cut into 1½-inch cubes	4 ounces		21	8
Onion, quartered	1	5	2	
Green pepper	1	2.5	1	
Cherry tomatoes	4			
Mushrooms	6			
		7.5	25	8

Calories: 1 serving—202

Alternate lamb cubes and vegetables on skewer. Brush cubes with barbecue sauce. Broil 4 inches from heat for 25 minutes, turning frequently.

Servings: 1
Exchange per serving: 3 low-fat meat, ½ vegetable

CHAPTER 9

Ground Meat Recipes

Meat Loaf Cake

Ingredients	Measure	Carbohydrates (gm.)	Protein (gm.)	Fat (gm.)
Ground beef	1½ pounds		126	144
Golden mushroom soup	1 can	20.4	8.7	10.5
Dry bread crumbs	½ cup	40	5	
Onion, chopped	¼ cup	2.5	1	
Egg, slightly beaten	1		7	5
Salt	½ teaspoon			
Pepper	generous dash			
Potatoes, mashed	2 cups	60	8	
Water	¼ cup			
		122.9	155.7	159.5

Calories: 1 serving—418

	20	26	26

Mix thoroughly beef, ½ cup soup, bread crumbs, onion, egg, salt, and pepper. Shape firmly into loaf and place in shallow baking pan. Bake at 350 degrees 1 hour. Frost loaf with potatoes and bake 15 minutes more. Blend remaining soup, water and 1 tablespoon of drippings. Heat and serve with loaf.

Servings: 6
Exchange per serving: 3 high-fat meat, 1½ bread

RECITE FOR

RECIPE FOR

Spaghetti Meat Loaf

Ingredients	Measure	Carbohydrates (gm.)	Protein (gm.)	Fat (gm.)
Ground beef	1½ pounds		126	144
Onion, chopped	½ cup	5	2	
Egg, slightly beaten	1		7	5
Salt, seasoned	1 teaspoon			
Spaghetti in tomato sauce	1 15¼-ounce can	46.8	9.6	2.1
		51.8	144.6	151.1

Calories: 1 serving—357

	9	24	25

Toss together all ingredients with a fork until combined. Turn into lightly greased loaf pan and bake, uncovered, 1 hour at 350 degrees.

Servings: 6
Exchange per serving: 3 high-fat meat, 1 bread

83

RECIPE FOR

Ribbon Meat Loaf

Ingredients	Measure		Carbohydrates (gm.)	Protein (gm.)	Fat (gm.)
Ground beef	1½	pounds		126	144
Egg	1			7	5
Catsup	2	tablespoons	9.8	.8	
Salt	2	teaspoons			
Dry mustard	1	teaspoon			
Pepper		dash			
Onion, chopped	¼	cup	2.5	1	
Margarine	2	tablespoons			30
Lemon juice	½	teaspoon			
Mushroom stems and pieces	1	4-ounce can	2.5	1	
Chopped parsley	2	tablespoons			
Thyme	¼	teaspoon			
Soft bread crumbs	4	slices	60	8	
			74.8	143.8	179
Calories: 1 serving—414			12	24	30

Combine beef, egg, catsup, 1½ teaspoons salt, mustard, and pepper in a large bowl; mix lightly with a fork just until blended. Saute onion in margarine just until soft; remove from heat. Stir in lemon juice, mushroom, parsley, ½ teaspoon salt, and thyme. Pour over bread crumbs; toss lightly to mix. Spoon half of meat mixture in greased loaf pan; top with stuffing; pat remaining meat mixture over stuffing to cover completely. Bake at 350 degrees for 1 hour.

Servings: 6
Exchange per serving: 3 high-fat meat, 1 bread, 1 fat

Cheese-Filled Meat Loaf

Ingredients	Measure	Car-bohy-drates (gm.)	Pro-tein (gm.)	Fat (gm.)
Ground beef	1½ pounds		126	144
Tomato sauce	16 ounces	56	16	
Egg, lightly beaten	1		7	5
Dry bread crumbs	½ cup	40	5	
Onion, finely chopped	¼ cup	2.5	1	
Salt	1 teaspoon			
Pepper	¼ teaspoon			
Thyme	¼ teaspoon			
American processed cheese	6 ½-ounce slices		21	9
		98.5	176	158

Calories: 1 serving—316   12   22   20

Combine beef, half the tomato sauce, egg, bread crumbs, onion, and seasonings. Place half the mixture in loaf pan. Arrange 4 cheese slices on top and pack remaining meat evenly over the cheese layer. Turn out onto a shallow baking pan. Cut remaining cheese slices in strips and arrange on top of loaf. Bake at 350 degrees for 40 minutes. Pour remaining tomato sauce over loaf. Bake 30 minutes longer.

Servings: 8
Exchange per serving: 1 bread, 2 high-fat meat, 1 low-fat meat

Favorite Meat Loaf

Ingredients	Measure	Carbohydrates (gm.)	Protein (gm.)	Fat (gm.)
Eggs	2		14	10
Catsup	⅓ cup	24.5	2	
Warm water	¾ cup			
Onion soup mix	1 envelope	30	4	
Dry bread crumbs	1½ cups	120	16	
Ground beef	2 pounds		168	192
		174.5	204	202
Calories: 1 serving—417		22	26	25

Beat eggs lightly in large bowl. Stir in catsup, water, and soup mix. Add bread crumbs and beef. Pack into loaf pan. Bake at 350 degrees for 1 hour.

Servings: 8

Exchange per serving: 1½ bread, 3 high-fat meat

RECIPE FOR

Pizza Burger

Ingredients	Measure	Car-bohy-drates (gm.)	Pro-tein (gm.)	Fat (gm.)
Tomato soup	1 10½-ounce can	37	4	5
Ground beef	1½ pounds		126	144
Dry bread crumbs	¼ cup	20	3	
Minced onion	¼ cup	2.5	1	
Egg, slightly beaten	1		7	5
Salt	1 teaspoon			
Crushed oregano	⅛ teaspoon			
Mozzarella cheese, sliced	4 ounces		28	22
		59.5	169	176
		10	28	9

Calories: 1 serving—413

Combine ¼ cup soup with beef, bread crumbs, onion, egg, salt, and oregano. Place a square of foil on cookie sheet and pat meat mixture out on foil into a 10-inch circle forming 1-inch standing rim around edge. Spread remaining soup over meat. Top with cheese and more oregano. Can also add mushrooms. Bake at 450 degrees for 15 minutes or until done.

Servings: 6
Exchange per serving: 1 bread, 3 high-fat meat, ½ low-fat meat

Hasty Italian Pizza Supper

Ingredients	Measure	Carbohydrates (gm.)	Protein (gm.)	Fat (gm.)
English muffins, split	2	60	8	
Tomato, sliced	1	5	2	
Ground beef	½ pound		42	48
Onion, chopped	½ tablespoon			
Garlic, minced	¼ teaspoon			
Salt	½ teaspoon			
Mozzarella cheese	4 1-ounce sliced		28	22
Basil	⅛ teaspoon			
Oregano	⅛ teaspoon			
		65	80	70
		16	20	18

Calories: 1 serving—306

Toast split muffins lightly. Place halves on cookie sheet and top each with tomato slice. Combine beef, onion, garlic, and salt and blend well. Spread ¼ of mixture on top of each tomato slice. Top with slice of cheese and sprinkle with basil and oregano. Bake 15 minutes at 400 degrees.

Servings: 4

Exchange per serving: 1 bread, 1 low-fat meat, 2 high-fat meat

Pizza Buns

Ingredients	Measure	Car-Bohy-drates (gm.)	Pro-tein (gm.)	Fat (gm.)
Ground beef	1 pound		84	96
Tomato paste	1 can	42	12	
Salt	½ teaspoon			
Pepper	a few grains			
Hamburger buns	8	240	32	
Mushroom stems and pieces	1 4-ounce can	2.5	1	
Oregano	as desired			
Mozzarella cheese, sliced	8 ounces		56	44
		284.5	185	140
		36	23	18

Calories: 1 serving—398

Lightly brown meat in skillet. Stir in tomato paste, salt, and pepper. Toast buns slightly on cut sides. Spoon beef mixture on bottom half of buns; top with a spoonful of mushrooms, a sprinkle of oregano, and a slice of cheese. Place top of bun over filling. Wrap each bun securely in heavy foil. Heat in oven at 400 degrees for 15 minutes.

Servings: 8
Exchange per serving: 2 high-fat, 2½ bread

Chili Con Carne

Ingredients	Measure	Car-bohy-drates (gm.)	Pro-tein (gm.)	Fat (gm.)
Ground beef	1 pound		84	96
Onion, chopped	¼ cup	2.5	1	
Clove garlic, minced	1			
Tomato sauce	8 ounces	28	8	
Kidney beans	2 cups	80	29	2
Liquid (from beans and water)	2 cups			
Chili powder	2 teaspoons			
Tabasco	¼ teaspoon			
Salt	1 teaspoon			
		110.5	122	98
Calories: 1 serving—461		28	31	25

Brown meat, onion, and garlic, stirring to break meat into pieces. Add remaining ingredients. Cook over low heat 1 to 1½ hours, uncovered. Stir occasionally. Add water, if needed.

Servings: 4

Exchange per serving: 2 bread, 3 high-fat meat

Potato Burgers

Ingredients	Measure	Car-bohy-drates (gm.)	Pro-tein (gm.)	Fat (gm.)
Potatoes, cooked and diced	2 cups	30	4	
Salt	1 teaspoon			
Pepper	¼ teaspoon			
Grated onion	1 tablespoon			
Chopped parsley	1 tablespoon			
Tomato sauce	8 ounces	28	8	
Ground beef	1 pound		84	96
		58	96	96
Calories: 1 serving—372		15	24	24

Brown beef in skillet. Combine potatoes, salt, pepper, onion, parsley, and ¼ cup tomato sauce. Add to meat and brown 5 minutes. Pour remaining tomato sauce over all, cover, and simmer 10 minutes.

Servings: 4
Exchange per serving: 3 high-fat meat, 1 bread

RECIPE FOR

Hobo Stew

Ingredients	Measure	Carbohydrates (gm.)	Protein (gm.)	Fat (gm.)
Onion, thinly sliced	1 cup	10	4	
Olive oil	¼ cup			60
Ground beef	1¼ pounds		105	120
Red kidney beans, drained	1 1-pound can	40	15	1
Worcestershire sauce	1 tablespoon			
Whole kernel corn, drained	1 1-pound can	32	4	1
Tomatoes	1 32-ounce can	40	16	
Tomato sauce	16 ounces	56	16	
Basil	as desired			
Dry mustard	as desired			
Salt	as desired			
Pepper	as desired			
		178	160	137

Calories: 1 serving—498

| | | 30 | 27 | 30 |

Cook onion in oil until golden. Add beef and cook, stirring with fork to break up meat, until browned. Add remaining ingredients and mix well. Cover and simmer 15 to 20 minutes.

Servings: 6

Exchange per serving: 2 bread, 3 high-fat meat, 1 fat

Spaghetti and Meatballs

Ingredients	Measure	Car-bohy-drates (gm.)	Pro-tein (gm.)	Fat (gm.)
Onions, chopped	2	10	4	
Olive oil	2 tablespoons			30
Tomatoes	1 29-ounce can	30	12	
Tomato sauce	8 ounces	28	8	
Chopped parsley	¼ cup			
Garlic salt	2½ teaspoons			
Pepper	¼ teaspoon			
Crushed red pepper	¼ teaspoon			
Tomato paste	1 8-ounce can	42	12	
Meatballs (recipe page 94)		25	117	125
		135	153	155

Calories: 1 serving—430 plus 70 for spaghetti		23	26	26

Cook onions in oil until yellowed. Add tomatoes, bring to a boil, and simmer, uncovered, for 20 minutes. Add remaining ingredients and simmer uncovered 2 hours longer, stirring occasionally. Serve over cooked spaghetti allowing ½ cup spaghetti, 2 meatballs, and 1/6 sauce per person.

Servings: 6
Exchange per serving: 1 vegetable, 1½ bread, 3 high-fat meat

RECIPE FOR

Meatballs

Ingredients	Measure	Car-bohy-drates (gm.)	Pro-tein (gm.)	Fat (gm.)
Ground beef	1¼ pounds		105	120
Onions, minced	1	5	2	
Chopped parsley	¼ cup			
Dry bread crumbs	¼ cup	20	3	
Egg	1		7	5
Garlic salt	2 teaspoons			
Pepper	½ teaspoon			
Oregano	½ teaspoon			
		25	117	125

Calories: 1 serving—283   4   19.5   21

Combine all ingredients and shape into 12 balls.

Servings: 6 (2 meatballs each)
Exchange per serving: 3 high-fat meat

Spaghetti Amore

Ingredients	Measure	Car-bohy-drates (gm.)	Pro-tein (gm.)	Fat (gm.)
Ground beef	1 pound		84	96
Onion, chopped	½ cup	5	2	
Oil	1 tablespoon			15
Cream of mushroom soup	1 10½-ounce can	23	5	26
Tomato soup	1 10½-ounce can	37	4	5
Water	1 soup can			
Cheese, shredded sharp processed	1 cup		28	32
Spaghetti, cooked, drained	½ pound	120	16	
		185	139	174
Calories: 1 serving—477		31	23	29

Lightly brown beef and onion in oil. Add soups and water; heat. Add ½ cup cheese and spaghetti. Pour into 3-quart casserole, top with remaining ½ cup cheese; bake at 350 degrees for 30 minutes.

Servings: 6
Exchange per serving: 2 bread, 3 high-fat meat, 1 fat

Lasagne

Ingredients	Measure	Car-bohy-drates (gm.)	Pro-tein (gm.)	Fat (gm.)
Olive or salad oil	2 tablespoons			30
Onion, chopped	1	5	2	
Ground beef	1 pound		84	96
Garlic salt	2 teaspoons			
Pepper	¼ teaspoon			
Tomato paste	2 6-ounce cans	84	14	
Hot water	3 cups			
Lasagne noodles, cooked, drained	½ pound	120	16	
Cottage cheese	½ pound		28	12
Mozzarella cheese	½ pound		56	44
		209	200	182
Calories: 1 serving—411		26	25	23

Saute onion in oil. Add beef and cook and stir until crumbly. Mix in garlic salt, pepper, and tomato paste blended with hot water. Simmer, uncovered, 30 minutes. In shallow baking dish put a thin layer of sauce, half the noodles, all the cottage cheese, and thin slice of mozzarella. Repeat with half the remaining sauce, the noodles, the last of the sauce, and mozzarella. Bake at 350 degrees for 30 minutes. Leave out of oven for 15 minutes; then cut into squares.

Servings: 8
Exchange per serving: 2 bread, 2 high-fat meat, 1 medium-fat meat

Five-Layer Dinner

Ingredients	Measure	Car-bohy-drates (gm.)	Pro-tein (gm.)	Fat (gm.)
Potatoes, sliced, raw	4	60	8	
Ground beef	1 pound		84	96
Onions, sliced	2 cups	20	8	
Corn, drained	1⅓ cups	60	8	
Tomatoes	1 16-ounce can	20	8	
Salt	2 teaspoons			
Pepper	¼ teaspoon			
		160	116	96
Calories: 1 serving—492		40	29	24

In a casserole, layer potatoes, then beef, onions, corn, and tomatoes. Season layers with 2 teaspoons salt and ¼ teaspoon pepper. Bake at 350 degrees for 2 hours.

Servings: 4
Exchange per serving: 3 high-fat meat, 2½ bread

Stuffed Cabbage Rolls

Ingredients	Measure	Carbohydrates (gm.)	Protein (gm.)	Fat (gm.)
Cabbage leaves	12 large			
Ground beef	1¼ pounds		105	120
Salt	2 teaspoons			
Pepper	½ teaspoon			
Rice, cooked	1 cup	30	4	
Onion, chopped	1	5	2	
Egg	1		7	5
Poultry seasoning	½ teaspoon			
Tomato sauce	16 ounces	48	16	
Water	¼ cup			
Lemon juice	1 tablespoon			
		83	134	125
Calories: 1 serving—333		14	22	21

Cover head of cabbage with boiling water and let stand 5 minutes. Peel off 12 nice leaves. Combine beef, salt, pepper, rice, onion, egg, and poultry seasoning. Place equal portions in center of each leaf; fold sides of leaf over meat and roll up. Place in small casserole. Combine water, lemon juice, and tomato sauce and pour over rolls. Cover. Bake at 350 degrees for 1 hour.

Servings: 6 (2 rolls each)
Exchange per serving: 3 high-fat meat, 1 bread

RECIPE FOR

Meat Patty With Cheese Sauce

Ingredients	Measure	Car- bohy- drates (gm.)	Pro- tein (gm.)	Fat (gm.)
Ground beef	1 pound		84	96
Cream of celery soup, undiluted	1 10½-ounce can	19	4	12
Grated cheese	4 ounces		28	12
		19	116	120
Calories: 1 serving—406		5	29	30

Form beef into 4 patties and broil on both sides. Heat soup in double boiler and stir in cheese. As soon as cheese melts, pour ¼ sauce over each patty and serve at once.

Servings: 4
Exchange per serving: ½ bread, 1 low-fat meat, 3 high-fat meat

Oven Beef Bake

Ingredients	Measure	Car-bohy-drates (gm.)	Pro-tein (gm.)	Fat (gm.)
Elbow macaroni, cooked and drained	8 ounces	120	16	
Carrots, sliced	1 pound can	28	8	
Mushrooms, sliced	1 6-ounce can	3.5	1	
Ground beef	2 pounds		168	192
Onion, chopped	1	5	2	
Celery, thinly sliced	2 cups	20	8	
Margarine	4 tablespoons			60
Flour	5 tablespoons	30	4	
Salt	1 teaspoon			
Pepper	¼ teaspoon			
Condensed beef broth	1 10½-ounce can			
		206.5	207	252
Calories: 1 serving—496		26	26	32

Drain liquids from carrots and mushrooms and set aside. Combine vegetables with macaroni in a greased 12-cup baking dish. Brown ground meat and stir into vegetable mixture. Saute onion and celery in margarine until golden in same frying pan; sprinkle with flour, salt, and pepper, then stir in. Cook, stirring constantly, just until bubbly. Combine beef broth with saved vegetable juices; add water, if needed, to make 3 cups; stir into onion mixture. Continue cooking and stirring until sauce thickens and boils 1 minute. Pour over meat and vegetables; cover. Bake at 350 for 1 hour.

Servings: 8
Exchange per serving: 2 bread, 3 high-fat meat, 1 fat

Meat Roll

Ingredients	Measure	Car-bohy-drates (gm.)	Pro-tein (gm.)	Fat (gm.)
Eggs, beaten	2		14	10
Soft bread crumbs	¾ cup	60	8	
Tomato juice	½ cup	5	2	
Parsley	2 tablespoons			
Oregano	½ teaspoon			
Worcestershire sauce	1 tablespoon			
Salt	¼ teaspoon			
Pepper	¼ teaspoon			
Garlic clove, minced	1 small			
Ground beef	2 pounds		168	192
Thin slices boiled ham	Eight 1 ounce		56	44
Mozzarella cheese, shredded	6 ounces		42	33
Mozzarella cheese, slices	Three 1 ounce		21	16.5
		65	311	296
Calories: 1 serving—520		8	39	37

Combine first 10 ingredients and pat onto wax paper into a 12 × 10-inch rectangle. Arrange ham slices on top, leaving half-inch margin around edges. Sprinkle shredded cheese over ham. Starting from short edge, roll up meat, using wax paper to lift. Seal edges and ends. Place roll, seam side down, in 13 × 9 × 2-inch baking pan. Bake 350 degrees for 1¼ hours. Place halved cheese slices on top and bake additional 5 minutes. Let set 5 minutes before serving.

Servings: 8
Exchange per serving: ½ bread, 2½ medium-fat meat, 3 high-fat meat

Stuffed Eggplant

Ingredients	Measure	Carbohy-drates (gm.)	Pro-tein (gm.)	Fat (gm.)
Eggplant, cut in half lengthwise	1 small	10	4	
Ground beef	½ pound		42	48
Onion, chopped	¼ cup	2.5	1	
Salt	1 teaspoon			
Garlic powder	¼ teaspoon			
Pepper	¼ teaspoon			
Flour	1 tablespoon	6	.8	
Milk, skim	½ cup	6	4	
Swiss cheese, shredded	½ cup		28	12
		24.5	74.8	60
Calories: 1 serving—479		12	40	30

Preheat oven to 350°. Scoop out pulp of eggplant, leaving shell half-inch thick. Dice pulp. Brown ground beef and drain. Add onion, salt, garlic, pepper, and diced eggplant. Cover and simmer 15 minutes. Blend in flour; stir in milk. Stir over medium heat about 1 minute, until mixture thickens. Blend in ¼ cup cheese. Fill eggplant shells with meat mixture; top with remaining cheese. Cook 20 minutes, or until eggplant is tender.

Servings: 2
Exchange per serving: 1 vegetable, ½ bread, 3 high-fat meat, 2 low-fat meat

Meat-Onion-Potato Casserole

Ingredients	Measure	Carbohydrates (gm.)	Protein (gm.)	Fat (gm.)
Onions, sliced	2 large	10	4	
Artificial sweetener =	1 teaspoon sugar			
Margarine	1 tablespoon			15
Potatoes, mashed	3 cups	90	12	
Pot roast or roast beef, slices	Eight 2-ounce slices		112	88
Green peas, frozen	1 cup	30	4	
Gravy	1 10½-ounce can	15	9	6
Parmesan cheese, grated	2 tablespoons		5	4
Paprika	½ teaspoon			
		145	146	113
Calories: 1 serving—273		18	18	14

Place onions in hot, dry skillet; sprinkle with artificial sweetener and stir fry until onions start to brown. Add margarine and cook until onions are tender, stirring occasionally. Remove from heat. Spread half of mashed potatoes in greased 2-quart shallow baking dish. Arrange meat on top, then onions, peas, and gravy. Cover with remaining mashed potatoes and sprinkle with parmesan and paprika. Bake at 375 degrees for 35 minutes.

Servings: 8
Exchange per serving: 1½ bread, 2 medium-fat meat, ½ fat

Spaghetti Pie

Ingredients	Measure	Car-bohy-drates (gm.)	Pro-tein (gm.)	Fat (gm.)
Spaghetti, cooked and drained	6 ounces	90	12	
Margarine	2 tablespoons			30
Parmesan cheese	5 tablespoons		12.5	10
Eggs, beaten	2		14	10
Ground beef	1 pound		84	96
Onion	1 medium	5	2	
Green pepper, chopped	½			
Whole tomatoes, cut in pieces	1 8-ounce can	10	4	
Tomato paste	1 6-ounce can	42	7	
Artificial sweetener =	1 teaspoon sugar			
Oregano	1 teaspoon			
Garlic	1 clove			
Salt	½ teaspoon			
Pepper	dash			
Cottage cheese	1 cup		28	12
Mozzarella cheese, shredded	4 ounces		28	22
		147	191.5	180
Calories: 1 serving—372		18	24	23

Mix spaghetti while hot with margarine, parmesan cheese, and eggs. Spread over bottom and up sides of buttered 10-inch pie pan. Cook ground meat until it loses red color. Add onion and green pepper and cook until tender. Drain grease. Add tomatoes and their liquid, tomato paste, artificial sweetener, oregano, garlic, salt, and pepper. Cook until hot. Spread cottage cheese over spaghetti. Spoon meat mixture on top. Bake uncovered at 350 degrees for 20 minutes. Sprinkle mozzarella on top. Bake 5 minutes more. Let stand 5 minutes.

Servings: 8
Exchange per serving: ¼ vegetable, 1 bread, 3 high-fat meat

CHAPTER 10

Poultry Recipes

RECIPE FOR

Chicken Paella

Ingredients	Measure	Carbohydrates (gm.)	Protein (gm.)	Fat (gm.)
Onions, sliced	1 medium	5	2	
Green pepper, chopped	½ cup	5	2	
Monosodium glutamate	2 teaspoons			
Boiling water	2½ cups			
Converted rice	1 cup	120	16	
Margarine	¼ cup			60
Mushrooms, sliced	1 cup	10	4	
Green peas, frozen	1 10-ounce package	45	6	
Chicken, diced and cooked	2 cups		112	48
Tomato, cut in wedges	1 medium			
		185	147	108
Calories: 1 serving—382		31	24	18

Melt margarine in pan; sauté onion and green pepper; add mushrooms and sauté until tender. Add water, rice, and monosodium glutamate. Cover pan with lid and place in oven at 350 degrees for 25 minutes. Stir in peas and half the chicken. Arrange remaining chicken and tomato on top. Cover and return to oven for 15 minutes.

Servings: 6
Exchange per serving: 3 low-fat meat, 2 bread, 2 fat

Chicken Fricasee

Ingredients	Measure	Car-bohy-drates (gm.)	Pro-tein (gm.)	Fat (gm.)
Chicken broiler-fryer	3½ pounds		294	126
Onion, chopped	½ cup	5	2	
Carrot, pared and sliced thinly	1	2.5	1	
Celery, sliced thinly	1 stalk	1	.5	
Salt	2 teaspoons			
Peppercorns	6 whole			
Bay leaf	1			
Water				
Margarine	6 tablespoons			90
Flour	6 tablespoons	36	5	
Peas, frozen	1 10-ounce package	45	6	
Cornmeal dumplings (recipe page 112)				
		89.5	308.5	216
Calories: 1 serving—443		11	39	27

110

Combine first 7 ingredients in Dutch oven with water to cover. Heat to boiling, cover, and simmer 2 hours, or until chicken is tender. Remove and set aside. Strain broth into 4-cup measure (add water, if necessary, to make 4 cups). Press vegetables through sieve into broth. Melt margarine in same kettle; stir in flour; cook, stirring constantly, just until bubbly. Stir in 4 cups broth; continue cooking and stirring until gravy thickens and boils 1 minute. Season to taste with salt and pepper. Place chicken in gravy, add peas, and heat slowly to boiling while preparing cornmeal dumplings. Drop batter in 8 mounds on top of boiling chicken; cover. Cook until puffy light, about 20 minutes.

Servings: 8
Exchange per serving: 1 bread, 5 low-fat meat, 2 fat plus 1 bread, 1 fat for dumplings

RECIPE FOR

Cornmeal Dumplings

Ingredients	Measure	Carbohydrates (gm.)	Protein (gm.)	Fat (gm.)
Flour, sifted	¾ cup	72	10	
Baking powder	1½ teaspoons			
Salt	½ teaspoon			
Yellow cornmeal	½ cup	60	8	
Milk, skim	⅔ cup	8	6	
Vegetable oil	2 tablespoons			30
		140	24	30

Calories: 1 serving—117   18   3   3.7

Place dry ingredients in a bowl. Combine milk and oil in 1-cup measure and add all at once to dry ingredients. Stir just until evenly moist. (Dough will be soft.)

Servings: 8
Exchange per serving: 1 bread, 1 fat

Chicken Cacciatora

Ingredients	Measure	Car- bohy- drates (gm.)	Pro- tein (gm.)	Fat (gm.)
Chicken breasts, frying	3½ pounds		294	126
Olive oil	2 tablespoons			30
Garlic	1 clove			
Oregano	1 teaspoon			
Salt	as desired			
Pepper	as desired			
Sliced mushrooms	1½ cups	15	6	
Stewed tomatoes	1 16-ounce can	20	8	
Parsley	as desired			
		35	308	156
Calories: 1 serving—352		4	39	20

Brown chicken in oil with garlic. Before turning, sprinkle with oregano, salt, and pepper. Remove garlic. Add mushrooms, brown lightly. Add tomatoes. Cover and simmer 30 minutes. Uncover; continue cooking until sauce is reduced to consistency desired and chicken is very tender. Garnish with parsley.

Servings: 8
Exchange per serving: 1 vegetable, 5 low-fat meat, 1 fat

Oven Crisp Chicken

Ingredients	Measure	Car- bohy- drates (gm.)	Pro- tein (gm.)	Fat (gm.)
Chicken, broiler- fryer	3½ pounds		294	126
Onion soup mix	2 envelopes	60	8	
Dry bread crumbs	1 cup	40	5	
Salt	1 teaspoon			
Pepper	⅛ teaspoon			
		100	307	126
Calories: 1 serving—348		13	38	16

Combine soup mix, bread crumbs, salt, and pepper in a paper bag. Shake chicken pieces, a few at a time, in mixture to coat well. Place, not touching, in a single layer in a lightly oiled shallow baking pan. Bake at 350 degrees for 1 hour, or until chicken is tender and richly browned.

Servings: 8
Exchange per serving: 1 bread, 5 low-fat meat

Apricot Chicken

Ingredients	Measure	Car-bohy-drates (gm.)	Pro-tein (gm.)	Fat (gm.)
Apricot jelly, low calorie	1 8-ounce jar	15		
Onion soup mix	1 envelope	30	4	
Russian dressing, low calorie	1 8-ounce jar	56		1
Chicken, broiler-fryer	3½ pounds		294	126
		101	298	127
Calories: 1 serving—344		13	37	16

Combine jelly, soup mix and dressing. Pour over chicken and marinate 24 hours. Bake uncovered for 1½ hours at 350 degrees.

Servings: 8
Exchange per serving: 1 bread, 5 low-fat meat

Man's Barbecued Chicken

Ingredients	Measure		Car-bohy-drates (gm.)	Pro-tein (gm.)	Fat (gm.)
Garlic salt	2	teaspoons			
Pepper	¼	teaspoon			
Tomato juice	1½	cups	15	6	
Cayenne pepper	¼	teaspoon			
Dry mustard	¼	teaspoon			
Bay leaf	1				
Worcestershire sauce	4½	teaspoons			
Cider vinegar	¾	cup			
Artificial sweetener =	1	teaspoon sugar			
Margarine or salad oil	3	tablespoons			45
Chicken, broiler-fryer	3½	pounds		294	126
Onions	1½		7.5	3	
			22.5	303	171
Calories: 1 serving—353			3	38	21

Day before or early in day make barbecue sauce: combine 2 teaspoons garlic salt, ¼ teaspoon pepper, tomato juice, cayenne, mustard, bay leaf, Worcestershire, vinegar, artificial sweetener, and margarine. Simmer, uncovered, 10 minutes, then refrigerate. About 1½ hours before serving arrange chicken, skin side up, in shallow pan. Sprinkle lightly with salt and pepper. Slice onions and layer over chicken. Pour on sauce. Bake, uncovered, at 350 degrees for 30 minutes, basting often; turn, bake 45 minutes longer, basting often.

Servings: 8
Exchange per serving: 1 vegetable, 5 low-fat meat, 1 fat

Dieter's Chicken With Pineapple

Ingredients	Measure	Car-bohy-drates (gm.)	Pro-tein (gm.)	Fat (gm.)
Chicken, broiler-fryer	3½ pounds		294	126
Soy sauce	¼ cup			
Monosodium glutamate	1 teaspoon			
Lemon juice	2 tablespoons			
Clove garlic, crushed	1			
Sliced pineapple, dietetic	1 8-ounce can	40		
		40	294	126
Calories: 1 serving—312		5	37	16

Mix soy sauce, lemon juice, and garlic. Place chicken in shallow pan; sprinkle with monosodium glutamate; pour mixture over and let stand for a few hours, turning once or twice. Remove chicken to broiling rack (reserve marinade). Broil chicken 6 inches from fire for 20 minutes until charred. Turn. Drain pineapple (reserve juice) and place slices in pan under rack. Spoon marinade over pineapple. Continue broiling until chicken is charred and tender—about 10 minutes. Remove chicken and pineapple to serving dish. Remove rack, add pineapple juice to marinade, and stir over low heat. Serve sauce on side. (Can be spooned over cooked rice as a side dish.)

Servings: 8
Exchange per serving: 1 vegetable, 1 low-fat meat

Chicken Chow Mein

Ingredients	Measure	Carbohydrates (gm.)	Protein (gm.)	Fat (gm.)
Chicken bouillon cube	1			
Artificial sweetener =	2 tablespoons sugar			
Water	¾ cup			
Soy sauce	¼ cup			
Chicken, diced and cooked	3 cups		168	72
Chinese vegetables	1 16-ounce can			
Chinese noodles	1 can	45	6	20
Rice, cooked	2 cups	60	8	
		105	182	92
Calories: 1 serving—327		18	30	15

Combine bouillon cube, artificial sweetener, water, and soy sauce. Bring to a boil and simmer 5 minutes. Heat chicken in sauce. Heat Chinese vegetables. Combine with chicken and serve over rice and Chinese noodles.

Servings: 6
Exchange per serving: 1 bread, 4 low-fat meat, 1 fat

Chicken Pie—Using Leftover Chicken

Ingredients	Measure	Car-bohy-drates (gm.)	Pro-tein (gm.)	Fat (gm.)
Chicken, cooked	3 cups		168	72
Potatoes, quartered	6	90	12	
Onions, quartered	4	20	8	
Carrots, sliced	4	20	8	
Parsley, chopped	2 tablespoons			
Margarine	3 tablespoons			45
Flour	2 tablespoons	12	2	
Salt	½ teaspoon			
Pepper	⅛ teaspoon			
Chicken broth	1 13¾-ounce can			
Refrigerated biscuits	1 8-ounce package	150	20	
		292	218	117
Calories: 1 serving—520		49	36	20

In large covered saucepan cook potatoes, onions and carrots in 2 cups water for 15 minutes. Drain well. Mix with chicken and parsley in 3-quart baking dish. Blend flour, salt and pepper in 2 tablespoons melted margarine. Gradually stir in chicken broth and cook, stirring constantly, until sauce thickens and comes to a boil. Pour over chicken-vegetable mixture. Flatten biscuits and arrange over top of mixture. Brush with 1 tablespoon melted margarine. Bake 45 minutes at 350 degrees.

Servings: 6
Exchange per serving: 1 vegetable, 4 low-fat meat, 3 bread, 1½ fat

Potted Chicken

Ingredients	Measure		Carbohydrates (gm.)	Protein (gm.)	Fat (gm.)
Chicken, broiler-fryer, cut up	3½	pounds		294	126
Oil	2	tablespoons			30
Onion, chopped	½	cup	5	2	
Tomato sauce	8	ounces	28	8	
Water	¼	cup			
Garlic	1	clove			
Salt	1	teaspoon			
Paprika	½	teaspoon			
Pepper		dash			
			33	304	156
Calories: 1 serving—344			4	38	20

Brown chicken in oil in skillet. Set aside. Cook onion in drippings, drain excess fat, and stir in remaining ingredients. Return chicken, cover, and simmer 45 minutes or until chicken is tender.

Servings: 8
Exchange per serving: 1 vegetable, 5 low-fat meat, 1 fat

Orange Glazed Chicken

Ingredients	Measure	Car-bohy-drates (gm.)	Pro-tein (gm.)	Fat (gm.)
Chicken, broiler-fryer, cut up	3½ pounds		294	126
Onion soup mix	1 envelope	30	4	
Orange juice con-centrate, thawed	6 ounces	60		
		90	298	126
Calories: 1 serving—336		11	37	16

Preheat oven to 400 degrees. Combine soup mix and orange concentrate. Place chicken in shallow pan and brush with half soup/orange mixture. Bake 1 hour, basting frequently, or until chicken is tender.

Servings: 8
Exchange per serving: ½ fruit, 1 vegetable, 5 low-fat meat

Chicken 'n Ham Roll-Ups

Ingredients	Measure	Carbohydrates (gm.).	Protein (gm.)	Fat (gm.)
Boneless chicken breasts	1½ pounds		126	54
Boiled ham, slices	6 1-ounce slices		42	33
Margarine	2 tablespoons			30
Cream of chicken soup	1 10¾-ounce can	15	2	20
White wine	¼ cup	4	.2	
		19	170	137
Calories: 1 serving—332		3	28	23

Place chicken between two sheets of waxed paper and pound until thin and flat. Top with slice of ham, roll up, and secure with toothpicks. Brown in margarine, stir in soup and wine. Cover and cook over low heat for 20 minutes.

Servings: 6

Exchange per serving: ¼ bread, 3 low-fat meat, 1 medium-fat meat, 1½ fat

Chicken Casserole Dinner

Ingredients	Measure	Car-bohy-drates (gm.)	Pro-tein (gm.)	Fat (gm.)
Chicken, broiler-fryer, cut up	3½ pounds		294	126
Salt	1 teaspoon			
Pepper	¼ teaspoon			
Oil	2 tablespoons			30
Mushrooms, sliced	½ pound	5	2	
Onions, sliced	1	5	2	
Garlic, minced	1 clove			
Thyme	½ teaspoon			
White wine	½ cup	8	4	
Peas, thawed slightly	1 10-ounce package	45	6	
		63	304	156
Calories: 1 serving—359		8	38	20

Sprinkle chicken with half the salt and pepper. Brown in skillet; add mushrooms, onion, garlic, thyme, and second half of salt and pepper. Saute until mushrooms and onion are tender. Add wine, cover, and simmer 20 minutes. Stir in peas, cover, and simmer 10 minutes or until chicken and peas are tender.

Servings: 8
Exchange per serving: ½ bread, 5 low-fat meat, 1 fat

Fish Recipes

Scandinavian Fish Bake

Ingredients	Measure	Carbohy-drates (gm.)	Pro-tein (gm.)	Fat (gm.)
Cod, haddock, or flounder fillets	1 pound		84	36
Flour	4 tablespoons	24	3.2	
Salt	2 teaspoons			
Pepper	¼ teaspoon			
Milk, skim	1 cup	12	8	
Dry bread crumbs	½ cup	40	5	
Margarine, melted	2 tablespoons			30
Chopped parsley	1 tablespoon			
Sour cream	½ cup			20
		76	100.2	86
Calories: 1 serving—374		19	25	22

Cut fillets into serving pieces and coat with mixture of flour, salt, and pepper. Arrange in single layer in baking dish and pour milk over. Bake at 350 degrees for 45 minutes. Mix crumbs with margarine in a small bowl. Stir parsley into sour cream in another bowl. Remove fish from oven; spoon sour cream over, then buttered crumbs. Bake 10 minutes longer, or until sour cream is set.

Servings: 4
Exchange per serving: 1½ bread, 3 low-fat meat, 2½ fat

Broiled Cod Piquant

Ingredients	Measure	Car-bohy-drates (gm.)	Pro-tein (gm.)	Fat (gm.)
Cod fillets	1 pound		84	36
Mayonnaise	4 teaspoons			20
Salt	as desired			
Pepper	as desired			
Dry bread crumbs	¼ cup	20	2.5	
		20	86.5	56
Calories: 1 serving—234		5	22	14

Spread fish with mayonnaise. Sprinkle with salt and pepper. Broil 3 inches from fire for 8 minutes. Sprinkle with crumbs and broil 2 or 3 minutes or until browned.

Servings: 4
Exchange per serving: ½ bread, 3 low-fat meat, 1 fat

Fish Fillets in Mushroom Sauce

Ingredients	Measure	Car- bohy- drates (gm.)	Pro- tein (gm.)	Fat (gm.)
Fresh mushrooms	1 cup	5	2	
Margarine	3 tablespoons			45
Flour	2½ tablespoons	15	2	
Salt	½ teaspoon			
Cayenne	dash			
Milk, skim	2 cups	24	16	
Cod or haddock fillets	1 pound		84	36
Dry bread crumbs	¼ cup	20	2	
		64	106	81
Calories: 1 serving—352		16	27	20

Wash and slice mushrooms. Saute in margarine for 5 minutes. Add flour and seasonings, mixing to a smooth paste. Add milk gradually, stirring constantly. Cook until thickened. Place fillets in a baking dish and sprinkle with salt. Cover with sauce. Top with bread crumbs. Bake at 375 degrees for 30 minutes.

Servings: 4
Exchange per serving: 1 bread, 3 low-fat meat, 2 fat

Tomato Glazed Fillets I

Ingredients	Measure	Carbohy- drates (gm.)	Pro- tein (gm.)	Fat (gm.)
Vegetable or olive oil	2 tablespoons			30
Onion, thinly sliced	1	5	2	
Mushroom, stems and pieces	1 4-ounce can	2.5	1	
Cod or haddock fillets	1 pound		84	36
Garlic salt	½ teaspoon			
Salt	1 teaspoon			
Grated lemon rind	½ teaspoon			
Ground dill seed	¼ teaspoon			
Tomato juice	2 cups	20	8	
Flour	2 tablespoons	12	2	
Lemon juice	2 tablespoons			
Artificial sweetener =	2 tablespoons sugar			
Chopped parsley	1 tablespoon			
		39.5	97	66

Calories: 1 serving—289

| | 10 | 24 | 17 |

Saute onion in oil until tender. Add mushrooms. Arrange fillets over vegetables. Sprinkle with garlic salt, salt, lemon rind, and dill seed. Add tomato juice. Cover and cook over moderate heat for 10 minutes, until fish is easily flaked with a fork. Remove fish to heated platter. Blend flour and lemon juice together. Gradually add ½ cup of mixture from skillet. Pour back into skillet, stirring vigorously. Add artificial sweetener; cook over moderate heat, stirring constantly, until thickened. Pour over fish and garnish with parsley.

Servings: 4
Exchange per serving: 2 vegetable, 3 low-fat meat, 1½ fat

Yum Yum Sole

Ingredients	Measure	Car-bohy-drates (gm.)	Pro-tein (gm.)	Fat (gm.)
Sole or flounder fillets	1 pound		84	36
Flour	2 tablespoons	12	1	
Paprika	2 teaspoons			
Salt	1 teaspoon			
Salad oil	1 tablespoon			15
Margarine	¼ cup			60
Lemon juice	2 tablespoons			
Liquid red pepper seasoning	¼ teaspoon			
Parsley	a few sprigs			
		12	85	111
Calories: 1 serving—348		3	21	28

Mix flour, paprika, and salt; coat fish with this mixture. Place in greased shallow baking pan and brush with salad oil. Melt margarine in saucepan; add lemon juice and liquid red pepper seasoning. Broil fish 2 to 3 inches from fire for 8 minutes. Don't turn during broiling. Transfer to a warm platter and pour margarine mixture over the top. Garnish with parsley.

Servings: 4
Exchange per serving: 3 low-fat meat, 3½ fat

Paprika Fish

Ingredients	Measure	Carbohydrates (gm.)	Protein (gm.)	Fat (gm.)
Cod, haddock or flounder fillets	1 pound		84	36
Onion, sliced	1 large	5	2	
Margarine	2 tablespoons			30
Evaporated milk	¾ cup	18	12	15
Paprika	1 tablespoon			
Salt	¾ teaspoon			
Pepper	¼ teaspoon			
		23	98	81
Calories: 1 serving—304		6	25	20

Cook onion in margarine until golden. Put in shallow baking dish. Cut fish in 4 serving pieces and arrange on top of onion. Beat remaining ingredients together lightly and pour over fish. Bake in moderate oven (375 degrees) about 25 minutes.

Servings: 4
Exchange per serving: ½ milk, 3 low-fat meat, 2 fat

Luncheon Lobster

Ingredients	Measure	Carbohydrates (gm.)	Protein (gm.)	Fat (gm.)
Bay leaf	1			
Lemon, sliced	1			
Artificial sweetener =	1 teaspoon sugar			
Salt	1 teaspoon			
Rock lobster tails, frozen	3 8-ounce		90	38
Mushrooms	1 3-ounce can	2	1	
Flour	1 tablespoon	6	.6	
Milk, skim	½ cup	6	4	
Seasoned salt	½ teaspoon			
Soy sauce	½ teaspoon			
Egg yolk	1	.1	2.8	2.5
Parmesan cheese, grated	1 tablespoon	2	2	
		16.1	100.4	40.5
Calories: 1 serving—278		5	33	14

In saucepan combine 4 cups water, bay leaf, lemon slices, artificial sweetener and salt. Bring to boil. Add lobster tails and boil gently, 10 minutes. Drain.

Drain mushrooms and add water to make ½ cup. Stir into flour in small saucepan. Add milk, seasoned salt and soy sauce. Bring to boil, reduce heat and simmer 3 minutes.

In small bowl beat egg yolk and gradually stir in hot mixture. Return to sauce pan and cook, stirring, just to boiling.

Remove lobster from shells and cut into bite size pieces. (Keep shells intact.) Add lobster and mushrooms to sauce and heat through. Spoon into lobster shells and sprinkle with parmesan cheese. Broil 2 inches from heat 2-3 minutes, until cheese browns.

Servings: 3
Exchange per serving: ¼ milk, 4½ low-fat meat

Fish Stew

Ingredients	Measure	Car-bohy-drates (gm.)	Pro-tein (gm.)	Fat (gm.)
Onion, sliced	1	5	2	
Margarine	4 tablespoons			60
Catsup	1 cup	78	6	
Lime juice	2 tablespoons			
Bottled steak sauce	2 teaspoons			
Worcestershire sauce	dash			
Salt	½ teaspoon			
Pepper	⅛ teaspoon			
Frozen cod or sole, cut into serving size pieces	2 pounds		166	72
		83	174	132
Calories: 1 serving—277		10	22	17

Saute onion in margarine in heavy skillet or Dutch oven until soft. Add catsup, lime juice, steak sauce, Worcestershire, salt, and pepper. Bring to boil. Add fish, cover, and simmer 20 minutes.

Servings: 8
Exchange per serving: ½ fruit, 1 vegetable, 3 low-fat meat, 1½ fat

Ellie's Fish

Ingredients	Measure	Car-bohy-drates (gm.)	Pro-tein (gm.)	Fat (gm.)
Onion, minced	2	30	4	
Oil	1 tablespoon			15
Fish fillets	1 pound		83	36
Cream of mush-room soup	1 10¾-ounce can	30	4	20
Peas, cooked	1 10-ounce package	45	6	
		105	97	71
Calories: 1 serving—362		26	24	18

Saute onions and place in baking dish. Place fish over onions and bake at 350 degrees for 10 minutes. Pour heated soup over fish and bake an additional 8 minutes. Pour peas over top and bake a few additional minutes, until fish flakes.

Servings: 4
Exchange per serving: 2 vegetable, 1 bread, 3 low-fat meat, 1½ fat

Bouillabaisse

Ingredients	Measure	Car-bohy-drates (gm.)	Pro-tein (gm.)	Fat (gm.)
Stewed tomatoes	32 ounces	40	16	
Tomato sauce	16 ounces	56	16	
Potatoes, cubed	2 medium	30	4	
Onions, diced	2	10	4	
Green peppers, seeded and sliced	2	10	4	
Garlic cloves, minced	2			
Bay leaf	1			
Parsley, minced	⅓ cup			
Italian herb seasoning	1 teaspoon			
Salt	1 teaspoon			
White pepper	½ teaspoon			
Fish fillets, cut into large pieces (any firm fleshed fish)	2½ pounds		207	90
Shrimp, cooked	½ pound		56	24
Clams, chopped, undrained	6½ ounces		45.5	19.5
		146	353	134
Calories: 1 serving—266		12	29	11

Combine first eleven ingredients in 3-quart saucepan and bring to boil. Reduce heat, cover, and simmer 30 minutes. Add remaining ingredients and continue simmering about 10 minutes, until fish flakes easily with fork.

Servings: 12
Exchange per serving: ½ bread, 1 vegetable, 4 low-fat meat

Tomato Glazed Fillets II

Ingredients	Measure	Car-bohy-drates (gm.)	Pro-tein (gm.)	Fat (gm.)
Oil	2 tablespoons			30
Onion, sliced	1 medium	15	2	
Mushroom stems and pieces, drained	4 ounces	2.5	1	
Fish fillets	1½ pounds		124.5	54
Garlic salt	½ teaspoon			
Salt	1 teaspoon			
Lemon rind, grated	½ teaspoon			
Tomato sauce	2 cups	56	16	
		73.5	143.5	81
Calories: 1 serving—271		12	24	14

Heat oil in skillet; add onion and cook until tender. Add mushrooms and arrange fillets over vegetables; sprinkle with garlic salt, salt, and lemon rind. Add tomato sauce, cover, and cook over moderate heat for 10 minutes or until fish is flaked easily.

Servings: 6
Exchange per serving: ½ bread, 1 vegetable, 3 low-fat meat, 1 fat

Tuna and Salmon Recipes

Crown Tuna Casserole

Ingredients	Measure	Carbohydrates (gm.)	Protein (gm.)	Fat (gm.)
Margarine	¼ cup			60
Onion, chopped	½ cup	5	2	
Green pepper, chopped	1 cup	10	4	
Flour	2 tablespoons	12	1	
Tomatoes, canned	32 ounces	40	16	
Worcestershire sauce	1 tablespoon			
Dry mustard	1 teaspoon			
Salt	½ teaspoon			
Artificial sweetener =	½ teaspoon sugar			
Pepper	¼ teaspoon			
Tuna, water packed	1 7-ounce can		49	21
Buttermilk biscuits, refrigerator	1 8-ounce can	150	20	50
		217	92	131
Calories: 1 serving—402		36	15	22

In hot margarine sauté onion until limp, add green pepper and cook 5 minutes. Stir in flour until blended. Add tomatoes, Worcestershire, mustard, salt, artificial sweetener, and pepper; simmer, covered, 10 minutes. Add tuna and pour into 2½-quart casserole. Cut each biscuit into thirds and arrange with points up on casserole. Bake at 375 degrees for 25 minutes.

Servings: 6
Exchange per serving: 1 vegetable, 2 bread, 1½ low-fat meat, 3 fat

Salmon Croquettes

Ingredients	Measure	Car-bohy-drates (gm.)	Pro-tein (gm.)	Fat (gm.)
Salmon, drained	1 pound can		112	48
Dry bread crumbs	½ cup	40	5	
Eggs	2		14	10
Onion, chopped	2 tablespoons			
Salt	as desired			
Pepper	as desired			
Water	2 tablespoons			
		40	131	58

Calories: 1 serving—307   10   33   15

Combine salmon, ¼ cup bread crumbs, 1 egg, onion, salt, and pepper. Form into four patties. Beat other egg and add water. Dip patties in egg, coating well, and then in bread crumbs. Brown well on both sides in skillet.

Servings: 4
Exchange per serving: ⅔ bread, 4 low-fat meat, ½ fat

Salmon Puffs

Ingredients	Measure	Carbohydrates (gm.)	Protein (gm.)	Fat (gm.)
White bread, in pieces	4 slices	60	8	
Milk, skim	1 cup	12	8	
Eggs	4		28	20
Salt	¼ teaspoon			
Dry mustard	½ teaspoon			
Onion, sliced	1	5	2	
Salmon, drained	1 7¾-ounce can		54	23
		77	100	43
Calories: 1 serving—275		19	25	11

Combine all ingredients in blender. Cover and blend on high speed for 20 seconds. Pour into 4 buttered individual 10-ounce casseroles. Bake at 325 degrees for 30 minutes.

Servings: 4
Exchange per serving: ¼ milk, 1 bread, 3 low-fat meat, ½ fat

Salmon Pickle Loaf

Ingredients	Measure	Car-bohy-drates (gm.)	Pro-tein (gm.)	Fat (gm.)
Salmon, drained	1 pound can		112	48
Cream of celery soup	1 10¾-ounce can	19	4	12
Soft bread crumbs	1½ cups	120	16	
Dill pickles, chopped	½ cup			
Eggs, well beaten	2		14	10
Vinegar	1 tablespoon			
		139	146	70
Calories: 1 serving—221		17	18	9

Combine ingredients. Pack into greased loaf pan. Bake at 350 degrees for one hour. Let stand 10 minutes before unmolding.

Servings: 8
Exchange per serving: 1 bread, 2½ low-fat meat

Tuna Jambalaya

Ingredients	Measure	Car- bohy- drates (gm.)	Pro- tein (gm.)	Fat (gm.)
Margarine	2 tablespoons			30
Onion, chopped	½ cup	5	2	
Sliced mushrooms, drained	1 4-ounce can	2.5	1	
Tomato soup	1 10½-ounce can	37	4	5
Water	2 tablespoons			
Worcestershire sauce	1 teaspoon			
Pepper	a few grains			
Tuna, drained, water packed	1 7-ounce can		49	21

Instant rice, pre-
  pared according
  to package
  directions
	2 cups	60	8	

		67.5	64	56
Calories: 1 serving—258		17	16	14

Melt margarine in skillet. Add onion and mushrooms; cook about 5 minutes over moderate heat, until tender. Fold in soup, water, Worcestershire, pepper, tuna. Cook over moderate heat, stirring constantly, until heated. Serve over rice.

Servings: 4
Exchange per serving: 2 low-fat meat, 1 bread, 1 fruit, 1 fat

Tasty Tuna

Ingredients	Measure	Carbohydrates (gm.)	Protein (gm.)	Fat (gm.)
Cream of mushroom soup	1 10¾-ounce can	30	4	20
Milk, skim	¼ cup	3	2	
Peas, frozen, cooked and drained	1 10-ounce package	45	6	
Tuna, drained and flaked	1 7-ounce can		49	21
Croutons	½ cup	7	2	
		85	63	41
Calories: 1 serving—332		28	21	14

In saucepan blend soup and milk. Add peas and tuna. Heat, stirring occasionally. Garnish with croutons.

Servings: 3
Exchange per serving: 2 low-fat meat, 1½ bread, 2 fat

Tuna Miniatures

Ingredients	Measure	Carbohydrates (gm.)	Protein (gm.)	Fat (gm.)
Crushed corn flakes	2 cups	40	5	
Milk	⅓ cup	4	2.5	
Mayonnaise	¼ cup			60
Tuna, drained, water packed	1 7-ounce can		49	21
Parsley	1 tablespoon			
Lemon juice	1 teaspoon			
Worcestershire sauce	½ teaspoon			
Salt	¼ teaspoon			
Pepper	dash			
		44	57	81
Calories: 1 serving—280		11	14	20

Mix one cup corn flakes with milk and then mix in remaining ingredients. Form one-inch balls. Roll in remaining corn flakes. Bake at 425 degrees on well-greased cookie sheet for 15 minutes.

Servings: 4
Exchange per serving: ⅔ bread, 2 low-fat meat, 2 fat

Tuna-Rice Pie

Ingredients	Measure	Carbohydrates (gm.).	Protein (gm.)	Fat (gm.)
Instant rice	1 cup	60	8	
Water	1 cup			
Salt	1 teaspoon			
Margarine	1½ teaspoons			7.5
Eggs	3		21	15
American cheese	1 cup		56	24
Tuna, drained, water packed	1 7-ounce can		49	21
Milk, skim, scalded	¾ cup	9	6	
Nutmeg	⅛ teaspoon			
Pepper	⅛ teaspoon			
		69	140	67.5
Calories: 1 serving—239		12	23	11

Place rice in 9-inch pie pan. Bring water, ½ teaspoon salt, and margarine to a boil. Stir into rice, cover, let stand 5 minutes. Beat 1 egg slightly, blend into rice. Press against bottom and sides, not above rim, of pie pan. Sprinkle ½ cup cheese on rice crust. Top with half the tuna. Repeat with remaining cheese and then remaining tuna. Blend ½ teaspoon salt, 2 eggs, milk, nutmeg, and pepper. Pour over tuna. Bake at 400 degrees for 25 minutes. If desired, top with tomato wedges for last 5 minutes of baking.

Servings: 6
Exchange per serving: ⅔ bread, 3 low-fat meat, ½ fat

Seafood Salad

Ingredients	Measure	Car-bohy-drates (gm.)	Pro-tein (gm.)	Fat (gm.)
Crabmeat, tuna, or salmon	1 cup		28	12
Lemon juice	½ teaspoon			
Onion, finely minced	½ teaspoon			
Salt	as desired			
Paprika	as desired			
Celery, diced	½ cup	5	2	
Lettuce hearts, in small pieces	½ cup			
Mayonnaise	4 teaspoons			20
		5	30	32

Calories: 1 serving—214   2.5   15   16

Lightly mix first seven ingredients in order. Chill thoroughly. Just before serving toss with mayonnaise to moisten. Serve on crisp lettuce.

Servings: 2
Exchange per serving: 2 low-fat meat, 2 fat

RECIPE FOR

Tuna Mousse

Ingredients	Measure	Carbohydrates (gm.)	Protein (gm.)	Fat (gm.)
Unflavored gelatin	1 envelope		7	
Lemon juice	2 tablespoons			
Onion	1-inch slice			
Boiling water	½ cup			
Sour cream	½ cup			20
Mayonnaise	½ cup			60
Tuna, drained	14 ounces		98	42
Dill	1 teaspoon			
Paprika	¼ teaspoon			
			105	122

Calories: 1 serving—35   2   3

Place gelatin, lemon juice, onion, and water in blender. Blend. Add mayonnaise, tuna, dill, and paprika. Blend. Add sour cream. Blend. Place in 1-quart greased mold and chill for 24 hours. Serve as spread on crackers.

Servings: 40 tablespoons
Exchange per serving: ½ fat (be sure to add cracker exchange)

CHAPTER 12

Cheese and Egg Recipes

Deviled Eggs

Ingredients	Measure	Car-bohy-drates (gm.)	Pro-tein (gm.)	Fat (gm.)
Eggs, hard cooked	6		42	30
Mayonnaise	¼ cup			60
Worcestershire sauce	½ teaspoon			
Dry mustard	¼ teaspoon			
Salt	dash			
			42	90

Calories: 1 serving—163   7   15

Remove egg yolks and mash. Blend with remaining ingredients and spoon into egg-white shells.

Servings: 6
Exchange per serving: 1 medium-fat meat, 2 fat

RECIPE FOR

Cheese Soufflé

Ingredients	Measure	Carbohydrates (gm.)	Protein (gm.)	Fat (gm.)
Bisquick	¼ cup	19	2	4
Dry mustard	½ teaspoon			
Milk, skim	1 cup	12	8	
Grated cheese	1 cup		37	29
Eggs, separated	3		21	15
Cream of tartar	¼ teaspoon			
		31	68	48

Calories: 1 serving—136   5   11   8

Mix Bisquick and mustard in saucepan; add small amount of milk to make a paste. Stir in rest of milk gradually. Bring to a boil; boil 1 minute, stirring constantly. Stir in cheese. Remove from heat; stir gradually into egg yolks. Beat egg whites and cream of tartar until stiff. Fold in cheese mixture. Pour into ungreased 1½-quart baking dish. Set baking dish in pan of hot water (1 inch deep). Bake at 350 degrees 50 to 60 minutes, or until knife inserted near center comes out clean. Serve with mushroom sauce. (Recipe page 158.)

Servings: 6
Exchange per serving: ¼ milk, ¼ bread, 1 medium-fat meat, ½ fat

Cheese Blintzes

Ingredients	Measure	Car-bohy-drates (gm.)	Pro-tein (gm.)	Fat (gm.)
Filling: Cottage cheese	½ pound		28	12
Egg	1		7	5
Salt	¼ teaspoon			
Artificial sweetener =	¼ teaspoon sugar			
Cinnamon	⅛ teaspoon			
Flour	1 cup	96	12.8	
Milk, skim	1 cup	12	8	
Eggs	4		28	20
Salt	½ teaspoon			
Margarine, melted	1 tablespoon			15
Sour cream	8 tablespoons			20
		108	83.8	72
Calories: 1 serving—354		27	21	18

Combine filling and set aside. Sift flour and salt together. Beat eggs; add milk while beating. Gradually add flour. Heat small frying pan. (Teflon is perfect for nonfat cooking here.) Pour ¼ cup batter in pan and tilt to spread thinly. When edges brown and top bubbles, turn out onto clean towel, brown side up. Put 1 tablespoon filling in center and fold up. Place in lightly greased baking dish. Continue with rest of batter and filling. Brush tops with melted margarine and bake at 350 degrees for 30 minutes. Top each blintz with 1 tablespoon sour cream.

Servings: 4 (2 blintzes each)
Exchange per serving: ¼ milk, 1½ bread, 2 medium-fat meat, 2½ fat

Mushroom Sauce

Ingredients	Measure	Car-bohy-drates (gm.)	Pro-tein (gm.)	Fat (gm.)
Egg	1		7	5
Milk, skim	½ cup	6	4	
Lemon juice	1 teaspoon			
Parsley	1 teaspoon			
Onion	2 tablespoons			
Salt	½ teaspoon			
Pepper	dash			
Sliced mush-rooms, drained	1 4-ounce can	2.5	1	
		8.5	12	5
Calories: 1 serving—31		2	3	1.2

Put all ingredients into blender. Cover and blend on high speed for 10 seconds. Cook over simmering water in double boiler, stirring occasionally, for 10 minutes.

Servings: 4
Exchange per serving: ¼ milk

Creole Casserole

Ingredients	Measure	Carbohydrates (gm.)	Protein (gm.)	Fat (gm.)
Instant rice	1 cup	60	8	
Cheddar cheese, grated	2 cups		112	128
Tomatoes, with juice	1 19-ounce can	20	8	
Salt	1 teaspoon			
Onion, finely chopped	¼ cup	2.5	1	
		82.5	129	128
Calories: 1 serving—500		21	32	32

Spread ½ cup rice, right from the box, in a layer on bottom of greased 1½-quart baking dish. Cover with 1 cup of the cheese. Add remaining rice. Combine tomatoes and juice, salt, and onion in saucepan, crushing tomatoes and mixing well. Bring to boil. Pour over layers of rice and cheese. Bake, covered, at 350 degrees for 10 minutes. Remove from oven, uncover, spoon remaining cheese around edge of rice mixture, leaving center uncovered. Bake 5 minutes longer.

Servings: 4
Exchange per serving: 1 vegetable, 4 high-fat meat, 1 bread

RECITE FOR

RECIPE FOR

Baked Eggs

Ingredients	Measure	Car-bohy-drates (gm.)	Pro-tein (gm.)	Fat (gm.)
Egg	1		7	5
Milk, skim	2 tablespoons	1.5	1	
Salt	as desired			
Pepper	as desired			
Calories: 1 serving—83		1.5	8	5

Butter small custard cup lightly; spoon milk into cup. Break egg in cup; sprinkle with salt and pepper. Bake at 325 degrees for 20 minutes or until eggs are cooked as you like them. Serve in cups.

Servings: 1
Exchange per serving: 1 medium-fat meat

160

RECIPE FOR

Omelet

Ingredients	Measure	Carbohydrates (gm.)	Protein (gm.)	Fat (gm.)
Eggs, separated	4		28	20
Hot water	4 tablespoons			
Salt	as desired			
Pepper	as desired			
			28	20
Calories: 1 serving—146			14	10

Beat yolks till thick and creamy. Add water and seasonings. Beat egg whites until stiff but not dry, and fold into yolks. Pour egg mixture into heated pan (Teflon is perfect for nonfat cooking here) and cook over low heat until brown on bottom and dry on top. (Insert knife in center; if it comes out dry, omelet is done.) Fold over and turn on a heated platter.

You can insert any of the following fillings in center of omelet before folding over:

1. 3 spears cooked asparagus—free
2. ½ ounce grated cheese—½ meat exchange
3. 2 teaspoons dietetic jam or jelly—free
4. ½ ounce sauteed cubes of sausage—½ meat, ½ fat exchange
5. ½ ounce cooked meat or chicken—½ meat exchange

Servings: 2
Exchange per serving: 2 medium-fat meat

161

Cheese and Mushroom Ball

Ingredients	Measure	Carbohydrates (gm.)	Protein (gm.)	Fat (gm.)
Mushrooms, sliced, drained	1 4-ounce can	2.5	1	
Cream cheese, softened	8 ounces			80
Onion, finely minced	1 tablespoon			
Salt	½ teaspoon			
Worcestershire sauce	1 teaspoon			
		2.5	1	80

Calories: 1 teaspoon—14.4   1.6

Chop mushrooms. Mix into cream cheese with onion, salt, and Worcestershire sauce. Chill thoroughly. Shape into ball. Serve with assorted crackers.

Servings: 1 5-inch ball
Exchange per serving: 1 teaspoon—⅓ fat exchange

CHAPTER 14

Soups and Lunches

Quiche Lorraine

Ingredients	Measure	Carbohy-drates (gm.)	Pro-tein (gm.)	Fat (gm.)
Swiss cheese, shredded	8 ounces		56	24
Eggs	3		21	15
Milk, skim	1½ cups	18	12	
Salt	¾ teaspoon			
Pepper	dash			
Onion flakes	2 tablespoons			
Margarine	1 tablespoon			15
9-inch pie shell	1	96	14	81
		114	103	135
Calories: 1 serving—351		19	17	23

Spread cheese and onion flakes in bottom of pie shell. Beat milk, eggs, salt, and pepper in a bowl to blend. Pour into shell. Dot with margarine. Bake at 375 degrees for 40 minutes. Allow to stand 10 minutes.

Servings: 6
Exchange per serving: ¼ milk, 1 bread, ½ medium-fat meat, 1 low-fat meat, 3 fat

Chilled Pea Soup

Ingredients	Measure		Carbohydrates (gm.)	Protein (gm.)	Fat (gm.)
Frozen peas	20	ounces	90	12	
Artificial sweetener =	2	teaspoons sugar			
Onion, cut up	½		2.5	1	
Margarine	3	tablespoons			45
Flour	3	tablespoons	18	2	
Salt	2	teaspoons			
Pepper		dash			
Milk, skim	3	cups	36	24	
Water	2	cups			
Egg white, hard cooked, chopped	1		.2	3.3	
			146.7	42.3	45

Calories: 1 serving—196   24   7   8

Day before or early in the day, cook peas with salt, according to label. Drain, place in blender with onion; cover; blend smooth on high speed. In saucepan melt margarine; stir in flour, salt, and pepper; slowly stir in milk; then cook, stirring, until slightly thickened. Remove from heat and stir in pea mixture and water. Refrigerate. Serve cold, garnished with chopped, hard cooked egg white.

Servings: 6
Exchange per serving: ½ milk, 1 bread, 1½ fat

Chilled Tomato Creme Soup

Ingredients	Measure	Car-bohy-drates (gm.)	Pro-tein (gm.)	Fat (gm.)
Frozen cream of potato soup	½ of a 10¾-ounce can	15	4	6.4
Tabasco	dash			
Seasoned salt	2 teaspoons			
Horseradish	2 teaspoons			
Tomato, large, quartered	1	5	2	
Canned tomato juice	1½ cups	15	6	
Croutons	1 slice bread	15	2	
		50	14	6.4

Calories: 1 serving—86   13   4   2

Early in day combine all ingredients, except tomato juice and crouton, in blender. Cover, blend smooth on high speed. Add tomato juice, cover, blend 1 minute. Refrigerate. Stir soup well, pour into glasses. Top with a few croutons.

Servings: 4
Exchange per serving: 2 vegetable, ½ fat

Tomato Bouillon

Ingredients	Measure	Carbohy-drates (gm.)	Pro-tein (gm.)	Fat (gm.)
Beef bouillon	2 10¾-ounce cans			
Tomato soup	2 10¾-ounce cans	73.8	8.4	9.6
Basil	dash			
Water	3 soup cans			
		73.8	8.4	9.6
Calories: 1 serving—40.5		7.3	.8	.9

Combine all ingredients; simmer a few minutes.

Servings: 10
Exchange per serving: 1 vegetable

Egg Drop Soup

Ingredients	Measure	Car- bohy- drates (gm.)	Pro- tein (gm.)	Fat (gm.)
Condensed beef broth	1 10½-ounce can			
Water	2 soup cans			
Bay leaf	½ medium			
Egg	1		7	5
			7	5
Calories: 1 serving—13			1.1	8

Combine soup, water, and bay leaf. Bring to a boil. Beat egg slightly; slowly pour it in a thin stream into soup, stirring constantly. Remove bay leaf. Egg should form thin threads.

Servings: 6
Exchange per serving: free

Chicken Soup

Ingredients	Measure	Car-bohy-drates (gm.)	Pro-tein (gm.)	Fat (gm.)
Chicken pieces, stewing	3 pounds (including bone)			
Salt	4 teaspoons			
Water	3 quarts			
Celery	3 cups	30	12	
Onion, quartered	3	15	6	
Carrots	3 cups	30	12	
Pepper	6 cloves			

Combine all ingredients in a large pot; bring to a boil and simmer, covered, 4 hours. Remove chicken (can be used for chicken salad or chicken chow mein). Pour soup through strainer (reserve vegetables) and let stand so fat will rise to top; skim off fat.

Place ¼ cup cooked noodles in bowl; add ¼ cup cooked vegetables from soup; pour in ½ cup soup; top with knaidlach (recipe page 170).

Servings: 15
Exchange per serving: 1 bread, 1 fat, ½ vegetable (½ bread for noodles, ½ bread, 1 fat for knaidlach, ½ vegetable for vegetables)

Airy Knaidlach
(Dumplings for Chicken Soup)

Ingredients	Measure	Car- bohy- drates (gm.)	Pro- tein (gm.)	Fat (gm.)
Eggs	4		28	20
Matzo meal	1 cup	120	16	
Salt	1½ teaspoons			
Oil	4 tablespoons			60
Water	2 tablespoons			
		120	44	80

Calories: 1 serving—85.8   7.5   2.7   5

Early in day mix oil and eggs together. Add matzo meal and salt. Then add water. Refrigerate. Forty minutes before serving bring 3 quarts water to boil. Reduce flame so water bubbles slightly and drop in balls of mixture. Cover pot and cook 40 minutes.

Servings: 16
Exchange per serving: ½ bread, 1 fat

Pizza on English Muffins

Ingredients	Measure	Carbohydrates (gm.)	Protein (gm.)	Fat (gm.)
Onion, chopped	¼ cup	2.5	1	
Olive or salad oil	2 tablespoons			30
Tomatoes	1 19-ounce can	20	8	
Bay leaf	1			
Salt	1 teaspoon			
Artificial sweetener	= 1 teaspoon sugar			
Oregano	½ teaspoon			
Pepper	dash			
English muffins	4	120	16	
Mozzarella cheese	4 1-ounce slices		28	22
		142.5	53	52

Calories: 1 pizza—313		36	13	13

Brown onion in oil. Add remaining ingredients, except for muffins and cheese, cover, and cook slowly for 30 minutes. Stir occasionally. Split English muffins in half and place cut side up on cookie sheet. Spoon sauce on each muffin; top with ½ slice cheese. Bake at 450 degrees for 12 minutes.

Servings: 4 (2 pizzas per serving)
Exchange per serving: 1 vegetable, 2 bread, 1 medium-fat meat, 1½ fat

RECIPE FOR

Brunch Bake

Ingredients	Measure	Carbohydrates (gm.)	Protein (gm.)	Fat (gm.)
Onion, finely chopped	2 tablespoons	1.2	.5	
Margarine	¼ cup			60
Flour	¼ cup	24	3.2	
Salt	¼ teaspoon			
Pepper	⅛ teaspoon			
Milk, skim	2 cups	24	16	
Swiss cheese	3 ounces		21	9
Ham, diced	1 cup		56	44
Eggs, hard boiled, sliced	6		42	33
Bread cubes	¾ cups	30	4	
Margarine, melted	1 tablespoon			15
Bread, toasted	6 slices	90	12	
		169.1	154.6	161
Calories: 1 serving—457		28	26	27

Cook onion in margarine until tender but not brown. Blend in flour, salt, and pepper. Add milk slowly, stirring constantly. Cook and stir until thickened and bubbly. Add cheese and stir until melted. Place half egg slices in bottom of 8 × 8-inch baking dish. Sprinkle half the ham over the eggs and spoon half the sauce over both. Repeat layers. Bake at 350 degrees for 35 minutes. Toss bread cubes with melted margarine; sprinkle on top of casserole. Bake additional 15 minutes. Spoon over toasted bread.

Servings: 6
Exchange per serving: 2 bread, 3 medium-fat meat, 2 fat

Shrimp Toast

Ingredients	Measure	Carbohydrates (gm.)	Protein (gm.)	Fat (gm.)
Frozen shrimp, thawed	10 medium		14	6
Bread	2 slices	30	4	
Mayonnaise	¼ cup			30
American cheese, diced	2 1-ounce slices		14	6
Curry powder	dash			
		30	32	42
Calories: 1 serving—313		15	16	21

Cut bread in half diagonally and place on broiler pan. Place shrimp on bread in single layer. Mix mayonnaise, cheese and curry powder, and spread over shrimp. Broil 1–2 minutes 3–4 inches from heat or until topping starts to brown. Serve at once.

Servings: 2
Exchange per serving: 2 low-fat meat, 1 bread, 3 fat

CHAPTER 15

Sauces and Toppings

RECIPE FOR

Tangy Cocktail Sauce

Ingredients	Measure	Car-bohy-drates (gm.)	Pro-tein (gm.)	Fat (gm.)
Catsup	½ cup	39.2	3.2	
Parsley	1 teaspoon			
Horseradish	1 teaspoon			
Lemon juice	1 teaspoon			
Salt	½ teaspoon			
Worcestershire sauce	½ teaspoon			
Artificial sweetener =	2 teaspoons sugar			
		39.2	3.2	

Calories: 2 tablespoons—42.4   9.8   .8

Blend ingredients well. Chill to blend flavors. Excellent served as a dip for raw cauliflower.

Servings: Yield—½ cup
Exchange per serving: 2 tablespoons = 1 fruit

176

Hot Barbecue Sauce

Ingredients	Measure	Carbohy-drates (gm.)	Protein (gm.)	Fat (gm.)
Lemon juice	½ cup			
Tomato juice	¼ cup	2.5	1	
Salt	1 teaspoon			
Paprika	1 teaspoon			
Pepper	½ teaspoon			
Onion powder	½ teaspoon			
Margarine	1 teaspoon			5
Cider vinegar	⅓ cup			
Cold water	¼ cup			
Dry mustard	1 teaspoon			
Artificial sweetener	2½ teaspoons = sugar			
Red pepper	½ teaspoon			
Tabasco sauce	1 teaspoon			
Garlic powder	⅛ teaspoon			

Combine ingredients in saucepan and heat to boiling point.

Servings: 1½ cups
Exchange per serving: free

Polynesian Barbecue Sauce

Ingredients	Measure	Carbohydrates (gm.)	Protein (gm.)	Fat (gm.)
Tomato juice	1½ cups	15	6	
Soy sauce	½ cup			
Garlic, crushed	3 cloves			
Worcestershire sauce	1 tablespoon			
Hot pepper sauce	a few drops			
Lemon juice	1 lemon			

Combine all ingredients.

Servings: 2 cups
Exchange per serving: free

RECIPE FOR

Seafood Sauce

Ingredients	Measure	Car- bohy- drates (gm.)	Pro- tein (gm.)	Fat (gm.)
Mayonnaise	¼ cup			30
Catsup	¼ cup	19.6	1.2	
Parsley, minced	1 tablespoon			
Horseradish	1 teaspoon			
Onion, grated	1 teaspoon			
		19.6	1.2	30
Calories: 1 tablespoon—43.3		2.4	.1	3.7

Combine all ingredients, stirring until well blended. Serve over broiled fish fillet.

Servings: 8 tablespoons
Exchange per serving: 1 tablespoon = 1 fat

RECIPE FOR

Ruby Strawberry Sauce

Ingredients	Measure		Carbohydrates (gm.)	Protein (gm.)	Fat (gm.)
Strawberries, washed and hulled	1	pint	25		
Artificial sweetener =	32	teaspoons sugar			
Cornstarch	2	tablespoons	15	2	
Water	½	cup			
			40	2	
Calories: 1 serving—21			5	.3	

Slice half of strawberries and set aside. Mash other half in small bowl. Mix artificial sweetener and cornstarch in medium saucepan; stir in water and mashed strawberries. Cook, stirring constantly, until mixture thickens and boils 3 minutes. Strain into medium-size bowl; fold in sliced strawberries.

Serve warm or cold over ice cream, vanilla pudding, or slices of angel cake or pound cake.

Servings: 8
Exchange per serving: ½ fruit

Gelatin Whipped Cream

Ingredients	Measure	Carbohydrates (gm.)	Protein (gm.)	Fat (gm.)
Dietetic gelatin, any flavor	1 envelope			
Hot water	½ cup			
Light cream	1 cup			40
				40

Calories: 1 serving—45   5

Dissolve gelatin in hot water. Chill until slightly thickened. Add cream and beat until light and fluffy (about 1 minute). Chill several minutes to set slightly. Before using, stir until smooth and fluffy, like whipped cream. Serve on gelatin, cake, or pudding.

Servings: 2 cups
Exchange per serving: ¼ cup = 1 fat

Whipped Topping

Ingredients	Measure	Car-bohy-drates (gm.)	Pro-tein (gm.)	Fat (gm.)
Nonfat dry milk solids	¼ cup	12	8	
Ice water	¼ cup			
Artificial sweetener	=	4 teaspoons sugar		
		12	8	
Calories: 1 serving—20		3	2	

Combine ingredients and beat on high speed of mixer until consistency of whipped cream.

Servings: 4
Exchange per serving: ¼ milk

Pretend Sour Cream

Ingredients	Measure	Car-bohy-drates (gm.)	Pro-tein (gm.)	Fat (gm.)
Lemon juice	2 tablespoons			
Milk, skim	¼ cup	3	2	
Cottage cheese	1 cup		28	12
Salt	pinch			
		3	30	12
Calories: ¼ cup—63		1	8	3

Place lemon juice and milk in blender. Gradually add cottage cheese and salt, blending at low speed. Blend a few minutes at high speed until smooth. If mixture thickens on standing, thin with additional milk, but be sure to calculate the addition.

Servings: 1 cup
Exchange per serving: ¼ cup = 1 low-fat meat

Chocolate Frosting

Ingredients	Measure	Car-bohy-drates (gm.)	Pro-tein (gm.)	Fat (gm.)
Unsweetened chocolate	1 ounce	8	4	15
Evaporated milk, skim	6 tablespoons	18	6	10
Vanilla	½ teaspoon			
Artificial sweetener =	8 teaspoons sugar			
		26	10	25
Calories: 1 serving—43		3	1	3

Melt chocolate over hot water. Stir in milk. Mix well and cook until thickened, about 2 or 3 minutes. Remove from heat and stir in vanilla and artificial sweetener. If too thick, thin down with water.

Servings: 8
Exchange per serving: ¼ milk, ½ fat

Cream Cheese Frosting

Ingredients	Measure	Car- bohy- drates (gm.)	Pro- tein (gm.)	Fat (gm.)
Cream cheese	4 tablespoons			20
Dietetic pineapple or strawberry jam	2 teaspoons			
				20

Calories: 1 serving—45   5

Soften cream cheese at room temperature for 30 minutes. Add jam spread and beat vigorously with mixer. Spread on cake or cupcakes, allowing 1 tablespoon per serving.

Variations: To plain cream cheese add:

1. 1 tablespoon milk and artificial sweetener—1 teaspoon sugar, 2 drops vanilla
2. A few drops artificial coloring
3. ¼ teaspoon grated orange rind
4. ⅛ to ¼ teaspoon grated lemon rind

Servings: 4
Exchange per serving: 1 fat

CHAPTER 16

Desserts

Recipes calling for one envelope dietetic gelatin or pudding are based on envelopes yielding 2 ½-cup servings. (They would be made by using 1 cup of water or milk.)

If the envelope you use yields 4 ½-cup servings (made by using 2 cups of water or milk) use only one half the contents of the envelope.

Remember that dietetic gelatin can be used in place of regular gelatin and this opens up a wonderful area of light and low calorie desserts. The companies manufacturing regular gelatin often have recipes in magazine advertisements, and some offer small cookbooks with recipes utilizing their products. By substituting dietetic gelatin in these recipes you will have endless sources of dessert dishes. (Just be sure to calculate the additional ingredients that may be added and deduct them from your meal allowance.)

Apple Torte

Ingredients	Measure	Carbohydrates (gm.)	Protein (gm.)	Fat (gm.)
Apples	8	80		
Artificial sweetener =	1 cup sugar as desired			
Cinnamon	as desired			
Brown sugar	1 cup	240		
All-purpose flour	1 cup	96	12.8	
Butter or margarine, melted	¼ cup			60
Pecans, chopped	½ cup			40
		416	12.8	100
Calories: 1 serving—333		52	2	13

Peel and slice apples. Place in pan 2 inches deep; almost fill with apples (pack down tightly). Sprinkle with ¾ cup artificial sweetener and cinnamon to taste.

Topping: Combine brown sugar, flour, and butter or margarine until crumbly. Place on top of apples, pressing down to form a crust. Sprinkle with pecans. Bake at 375 degrees for 35 minutes, or until apples are tender and crust is firm.

Servings: 8
Exchange per serving: 1 bread, 4 fruit, 1½ fat

Graham Cracker Crust—8 or 9 inch

Ingredients	Measure	Car-bohy-drates (gm.)	Pro-tein (gm.)	Fat (gm.)
Graham crackers, crushed	1 cup (12 square)	90	12	
Margarine, melted	2 tablespoons			30
Artificial sweetener =	6 teaspoons sugar			
		90	12	30
Calories: ⅛ crust—88		11	2	4

Combine ingredients and press into 8- or 9-inch pan. Refrigerate 1 hour before filling.

Yield: 8- or 9-inch crust
Exchange per serving: ⅛ crust = ¾ bread, 1 fat

Rice Crispy Cereal Crust—8 inch

Ingredients	Measure	Car-bohy-drates (gm.)	Pro-tein (gm.)	Fat (gm.)
Rice crispy cereal, crushed	1 cup	20	2.6	
Margarine, melted	2 tablespoons			30
Artificial sweetener =	2 teaspoons sugar			
		20	2.6	30

Calories: ⅛ crust—44.5   2.5   .3   3.7

Combine ingredients and press into bottom of 8-inch pie pan. Chill while preparing filling.

Servings: 8-inch crust
Exchange per serving: ⅛ = ⅕ bread, 1 fat

Pastry (yields 14 tarts or 1 9-inch pie crust)

Ingredients	Measure	Car- bohy- drates (gm.)	Pro- tein (gm.)	Fat (gm.)
Water	¼ cup			
Flour	1¼ cups	120	16	
Salt	½ teaspoon			
Margarine	¼ pound			120
		120	16	120
Calories: 1 serving—121		9	1	9

Measure water, flour, and salt into small electric mixing bowl. Slice in margarine. Mix on low speed for 20 seconds. Shape into ball and roll out.

Tarts—cut into 14 circles and fit into tart molds. Prick with fork. Bake at 450 degrees for 10 minutes. Fill as desired.

Baked pie shell—fit into 9-inch pie pan. Prick with fork. Bake at 450 degrees for 10 minutes. Fill as desired.

Unbaked pie shell—fit into 9-inch pie pan. Fill as desired and bake according to filling directions.

Servings: 14

Exchange per serving: ⅔ bread, 2 fat (Be sure to calculate filling.)

Cool-La-La Lime Pie-Filling

Ingredients	Measure	Carbohydrates (gm.)	Protein (gm.)	Fat (gm.)
Eggs	2		14	10
Artificial sweetener	= ½ cup sugar			
Green coloring	a few drops			
Light cream	1 cup			20
Lime juice	⅓ cup			
Lime peel	1 teaspoon			
Vanilla ice cream	1 pint	60	8	40
		60	22	70
Calories: 1 serving—125		8	3	9

Beat eggs until thick and lemon colored. Slowly add artificial sweetener and continue beating until mixture is light and fluffy. Add green coloring, cream, lime juice, and grated peel. Mix well. Pour into freezing tray and freeze until firm. Whip vanilla ice cream until smooth and spread into crust. Turn lime mixture into bowl and beat smooth. Pour over ice cream. Freeze.

Servings: 8

Exchange per serving: ½ bread, ⅓ medium-fat meat, 1½ fat (Filling alone—add exchanges for crust you choose to make.)

Cherry-Cream Pie Filling

Ingredients	Measure	Carbohydrates (gm.)	Protein (gm.)	Fat (gm.)
Unflavored gelatin	1 teaspoon		7	
Milk, skim	1 cup			
	& 2 table-spoons	13.5	9	
Egg, well beaten	1		7	5
Artificial sweetener =	6 teaspoons sugar			
Salt	⅛ teaspoon			
Vanilla	½ teaspoon			
Sour pie cherries	1 1-pound can	60	4	1.6
Cherry juice	⅔ cup			
Cornstarch	2 tablespoons	15	2	
Artificial sweetener =	¼ cup sugar			
Almond extract	⅛ teaspoon			
Red food coloring	a few drops			
		88.5	29	6.6
Calories: 1 serving—65.6		11	3.6	.8

Soften gelatin in 2 tablespoons milk. In double boiler combine egg, 1 cup milk, artificial sweetener (=6 teaspoons sugar), and salt. Cook over boiling water, stirring constantly, until mixture coats a metal spoon. Add vanilla and softened gelatin. Chill until thickened but not set. Drain sour pie cherries, reserving ⅔ cup juice. Combine cornstarch, artificial sweetener (=¼ cup sugar), and cherry juice in saucepan. Blend well. Add cherries; cook over medium heat, stirring constantly, until mixture thickens. Remove from heat. Add almond extract and food coloring. Chill. Turn into crust. Spoon custard over cherries. Chill until firm, 4 to 6 hours.

Servings: 8
Exchange per serving: 1 fruit, ½ low-fat meat (Filling alone—
    add exchanges for crust you choose to make.)

Gelatin Cheese Torte Pie Filling

Ingredients	Measure	Carbohydrates (gm.)	Protein (gm.)	Fat (gm.)
Dietetic gelatin, any flavor	1 envelope			
Boiling water	½ cup			
Cream cheese	4 ounces			40
Artificial sweetener	= ¼ cup sugar			
Evaporated milk, whipped	6 tablespoons	18	6	10
		18	6	50
Calories: 1 serving—66		2	1.3	6.6

Dissolve gelatin in boiling water. Cool until it just begins to set. Cream together cheese and artificial sweetener. Add gelatin. Mix well. Whip milk according to package directions. Fold whipped milk into gelatin mixture. Pour filling into crust. Chill several hours or overnight.

Servings: 8
Exchange per serving: 1 fat (Filling alone—add exchanges for crust you choose to make.)

Chocolate Bavarian

Ingredients	Measure	Carbohydrates (gm.)	Protein (gm.)	Fat (gm.)
Unflavored gelatin	1 envelope		7	
Water	2 tablespoons			
Cocoa	¼ cup	14.4	2.4	6.4
Milk, skim	1 cup	12	8	
Artificial sweetener =	16 teaspoons sugar			
Vanilla	½ teaspoon			
Nonfat dry milk solids	1 cup	36	24	
Ice water	1 cup			
		62.4	41.4	6.4

Calories: 1 serving—41   5   3   1

Soften gelatin in water. Make paste of cocoa and milk. Heat over boiling water; add softened gelatin and artificial sweetener, stirring until gelatin dissolves. Remove from heat; add vanilla; and let stand until mixture thickens. Then combine milk solids and ice water; beat on high speed of mixer until consistency of whipped cream. Beat gelatin smooth and gradually add to the whipped milk. Spoon into oiled 6-cup mold. Chill until firm, about 3 hours.

Servings: 12
Exchange per serving: ½ milk

Cheese Pie

Ingredients	Measure	Car-bohy-drates (gm.)	Pro-tein (gm.)	Fat (gm.)
Low fat cream cheese	16 ounces			160
Eggs	3		21	15
Artificial sweetener, granulated =	⅔ cup sugar			
Almond extract	⅛ teaspoon			
Topping:				
Sour cream	1 pint			80
Artificial sweetener =	3 tablespoons sugar			
Vanilla	1 teaspoon			
			21	255

Calories: 1 serving—242   2   26

Beat cheese and add eggs, one at a time. Add artificial sweetener and extract and beat for 5 minutes. Pour into greased 9-inch pie pan. Bake at 325 degrees for 50 minutes. Cool 20 minutes. Spoon topping over top of pie. Bake 15 minutes. Cool and refrigerate.

You can also top the pie with a can of sour cherries mixed well with 1 envelope cherry dietetic gelatin. Be sure to add ½ fruit exchange to each serving for the cherries.

Servings: 10
Exchange per serving: 5 fat

Strawberry Whip

Ingredients	Measure	Car-bohy-drates (gm.)	Pro-tein (gm.)	Fat (gm.)
Strawberries, washed and hulled	1 pint	26		
Hot water	½ cup			
Dietetic straw-berry gelatin	2 envelopes			
Crushed ice	1¼ cups			
		26		

Calories: 1 serving—12   3

Wash and hull strawberries. Into an electric blender pour hot water, dry gelatin, and 1 cup of the strawberries. Cover; blend 30 seconds. Add crushed ice; blend 20 seconds longer. Add remaining strawberries. Blend about 3 seconds. Pour into chilled serving bowl. Chill 1 hour or until partially set. Spoon into serving dishes and garnish with mint, if desired.

Servings: 8
Exchange per serving: ⅓ fruit

Fruit Whip

Ingredients	Measure	Car-bohy-drates (gm.)	Pro-tein (gm.)	Fat (gm.)
Fruit juice, unsweetened*	1¾ cups	35		
Unflavored gelatin	1 envelope		7	
Artificial sweetener =	10 teaspoons sugar			
Salt	⅛ teaspoon			
		35	7	

Calories: 1 serving—41.6   8.7   1.7

Sprinkle gelatin over ½ cup fruit juice in saucepan. Cook over low heat, stirring constantly, until gelatin is dissolved. Remove from heat. Stir in artificial sweetener, salt, and remaining 1¼ cups fruit juice. Chill until thick but not set. Beat at highest speed until smooth and creamy. Chill until firm. Spoon into serving dishes.
*Orange, orange-grapefruit, apple, pineapple-orange, or pine-apple-grapefruit.

Servings: 4
Exchange per serving: 1 fruit

RECIPE FOR

Hawaiian Dessert

Ingredients	Measure	Car bohy- drates (gm.)	Pro- tein (gm.)	Fat (gm.)
Dietetic pineapple	6 slices	60		
Reserved juice	¾ cup			
Dietetic lime gelatin	2 envelopes			
Milk, skim	½ cup	6	4	
Almond extract	¼ teaspoon			
Crushed ice	¾ cup			
		66	4	

Calories: 1 serving—46.4   11   .6

Bring juice to a boil; add gelatin, stirring until gelatin dissolves. Combine pineapple and milk in blender; blend well. Add gelatin mixture, almond extract and ice. Mix thoroughly in blender. Pour into dessert dishes. Chill until set, about 1 hour.

Servings: 6
Exchange per serving: 1 fruit

Baked Custard

Ingredients	Measure	Carbohydrates (gm.)	Protein (gm.)	Fat (gm.)
Egg, lightly beaten	1		7	5
Artificial sweetener	3 teaspoons = sugar			
Milk, skim	1 cup	12	8	
Vanilla	½ teaspoon			
Nutmeg	as desired			
		12	15	5
Calories: 1 serving—76.5		6	7.5	2.5

Combine beaten egg with artificial sweetener; slowly add skim milk and vanilla, blending well. Pour mixture equally into two custard cups;* top with a sprinkling of nutmeg. Bake in pan of hot water in moderate oven, 325 degrees, about 1 hour or until mixture does not adhere to knife.
*If you rinse cups in cold water before pouring in mixture, custard will not stick.

Servings: 2
Exchange per serving: ½ milk, ½ medium-fat meat

Jellied Blanc Mange

Ingredients	Measure	Carbohydrates (gm.)	Protein (gm.)	Fat (gm.)
Unflavored gelatin	1 envelope			
Milk, skim	2 cups	24	16	
Salt	¼ teaspoon			
Extract	1 teaspoon			
Artificial sweetener =	8 teaspoons sugar			
		24	16	

Calories: 1 serving—40

6   4

Soften gelatin in ¼ cup cold milk. Dissolve in 1¾ cups very hot milk. Add artificial sweetener, salt, and extract. Pour into 2-cup mold or 4 individual molds. Chill until firm, about 2 hours.

This recipe can be made with any flavor extract—rum, butterscotch, fruit extracts, vanilla, etc. Sprinkle nutmeg on top when using vanilla. It can be whipped after chilling until syrupy (yields 6 servings), or it can be whipped when set and layered with dietetic gelatin.

Servings: 4
Exchange per serving: ½ milk

Eclairs

Ingredients	Measure	Carbohydrates (gm.)	Protein (gm.)	Fat (gm.)
Water	½ cup			
Margarine	4 tablespoons			60
Flour, sifted	½ cup	48	6.4	.4
Salt	⅛ teaspoon			
Eggs	2		14	10
Dietetic vanilla pudding	1 envelope			
Milk, skim	1 cup	12	8	
		60	28.4	70.4
Calories: 1 serving—198		12	6	14

Heat water and margarine to boiling in medium saucepan. Stir in flour and salt all at once with a wooden spoon; continue stirring until batter forms a thick smooth ball that follows spoon around pan. Remove from heat; cool slightly; beat in eggs, one at a time, until mixture is thick and shiny-smooth. Shape batter into 5 strips on ungreased cookie sheet. Bake at 400 degrees for 30 minutes until puffed and lightly golden. Remove at once from cookie sheet and cool completely on wire rack. Prepare pudding mix with milk and chill. Cut across each eclair and lift off top. Scoop out softened dough. Fill with pudding. Replace top. Put teaspoon of dietetic chocolate syrup on top.

Servings: 5
Exchange per serving: ½ milk, ½ bread, 3 fat

RECIPE FOR

Baked Alaska

Ingredients	Measure	Car-bohy-drates (gm.)	Pro-tein (gm.)	Fat (gm.)
Pound cake, 4 × 2¾ × ⅝ inches	4 slices	77.6	10	42.8
Ice cream, any flavor	1 pint	60	8	40
Egg whites	3	.6	9.9	
Cream of tartar	¼ teaspoon			
Salt	⅛ teaspoon			
Artificial sweetener =	6 tablespoons sugar			
Vanilla	⅛ teaspoon			
		138.2	27.9	82.8
Calories: 1 serving—351.9		34.5	6.9	20.7

Place ½ cup ice cream in custard cup to mold and turn out on piece of cake. Repeat with remaining cake and ice cream and place in freezer for 15 minutes. Beat egg whites with cream of tartar and salt at very high speed until soft peaks form. Gradually beat in artificial sweetener; add vanilla. Continue beating until egg whites form stiff peaks. Remove ice cream and cake from freezer. Spread meringue over both. Completely seal with the meringue. Return to freezer. Place heavy brown paper on cookie sheet and grease well. Preheat oven to 425 degrees. Place frozen Alaskas on cookie sheet and bake 5 minutes, or until delicately browned. Serve at once.

Servings: 4
Exchange per serving: 2½ bread, 4 fat

Pudding Surprise

Ingredients	Measure	Car- bohy- drates (gm.)	Pro- tein (gm.)	Fat (gm.)
Dietetic vanilla pudding	2 envelopes			
Milk, skim	2 cups	24	16	
Dietetic jam, jelly, or marmalade	8 teaspoons			
		24	16	
Calories: 1 serving—40		6	4	

Prepare pudding according to package directions using skim milk. Rinse 4 custard cups; place 2 teaspoons jam, jelly, or marmalade in each; pour in hot vanilla pudding; chill.

Servings: 4
Exchange per serving: ½ milk

RECIPE FOR

Frozen Dessert Shells

Ingredients	Measure	Carbohydrates (gm.)	Protein (gm.)	Fat (gm.)
Dream Whip	1 envelope	19.2	9.6	19.2
Cold milk, skim	½ cup	6	4	
Vanilla	½ teaspoon			
		25.2	13.6	19.2
Calories: 1 serving—41		3.15	1.7	2.4

Combine Dream Whip, milk, and vanilla and prepare as directed on package. Drop mixture onto wax paper, about ¼ cup at a time. With a spoon make a depression in the top of each mound. Freeze until firm, 2 to 3 hours. Fill shells just before serving.

Fillings:
1. ¼ cup fruit ice in each shell—add 1 fruit exchange
2. Cubes of dietetic gelatin—free
3. ¼ cup dietetic pudding—add ¼ milk exchange
4. ⅛ cup ice cream topped with dietetic chocolate syrup—add ¼ bread, ½ fat

Servings: 8
Exchange per serving: ¼ milk, ½ fat

Bread Pudding

Ingredients	Measure	Carbohydrates (gm.)	Protein (gm.)	Fat (gm.)
Bread, cubed	2 slices	30	4	
Eggs, slightly beaten	2		14	10
Artificial sweetener	16 teaspoons = sugar			
Vanilla	1 teaspoon			
Salt	⅛ teaspoon			
Milk, skim, scalded	2 cups	24	16	
Cinnamon	1 teaspoon			
		54	34	10
Calories: 1 serving—119		14	9	1.2

Place bread cubes in lightly greased 1-quart casserole. Combine eggs, artificial sweetener, vanilla, and salt and gradually add milk. Pour over bread cubes. Sprinkle with cinnamon. Place casserole in hot water in pan and bake at 325 degrees for 55 to 65 minutes.

Servings: 4
Exchange per serving: ½ milk, ½ bread, ½ medium-fat meat

RECIPE FOR

Parfait Royale

Ingredients	Measure	Carbohydrates (gm.)	Protein (gm.)	Fat (gm.)
Dietetic apple-raspberry sauce	15 ounces	52.5		
Dietetic vanilla pudding	2 envelopes			
Milk, skim	2 cups	24	16	
		76.5	16	
Calories: 1 serving—73.2		15.3	3	

Put 2 heaping tablespoons of sauce in each of 5 parfait glasses. Make pudding according to package directions and spoon evenly on top of sauce in parfait glasses. Let stand about 15 minutes until firm. Spoon remaining sauce on top of pudding. Refrigerate until chilled.

Servings: 5
Exchange per serving: 1 fruit, ½ milk

Chapter 17

Cakes

Spiced Cake

Ingredients	Measure	Carbohydrates (gm.)	Protein (gm.)	Fat (gm.)
Margarine	½ cup			120
Artificial sweetener	= ¼ cup sugar			
Eggs	2		14	10
Skim sour milk	1 cup	12	8	
Vanilla	1 teaspoon			
Flour	2 cups	192	26	1.8
Cinnamon	2 teaspoons			
Cloves	½ teaspoon			
Allspice	2 teaspoons			
Nutmeg	1 teaspoon			
Baking soda	1 teaspoon			
		204	48	131.8
Calories: 1 serving—136		13	3	8.2

Cream margarine with artificial sweetener. Add eggs. Combine dry ingredients. Add milk alternately with dry ingredients. Add vanilla. Pour into 8×8×2-inch pan. Bake at 350 degrees for 30 minutes. Cut into sixteen 2-inch pieces.

Servings: 16
Exchange per serving: 1 bread, 1½ fat

Coffee Crumb Cakes

Ingredients	Measure	Carbohydrates (gm.)	Protein (gm.)	Fat (gm.)
Flour	2 cups	192	26	1.8
Double-acting baking powder	3 teaspoons			
Salt	¾ teaspoon			
Cinnamon	¼ teaspoon			
Baking soda	¼ teaspoon			
Nutmeg	¼ teaspoon			
Margarine	½ cup			120
Milk, skim	1 cup	12	8	
Instant coffee	¼ teaspoon			
Egg, unbeaten	1		7	5
Artificial sweetener	= ½ cup sugar			
		204	41	126.8

Calories: 1 serving—115   11   2   7

Sift together flour, baking powder, salt, cinnamon, baking soda, and nutmeg. Cut in margarine until particles are fine. Reserve scant ¼ cup for topping. Combine milk, coffee, egg, and artificial sweetener. Add all at once to remaining crumb mixture. Stir 100 strokes with a spoon. Fill 18 muffin cups, lined with paper baking cups, half full. Sprinkle with reserved crumb topping. Bake at 375 degrees for 20 to 25 minutes.

Servings: 18
Exchange per serving: ⅔ bread, 1½ fat

Sponge Cupcakes

Ingredients	Measure	Car-bohy-drates (gm.)	Pro-tein (gm.)	Fat (gm.)
Eggs, separated	3		21	15
Salt	¼ teaspoon			
Cream of tartar	¼ teaspoon			
Artificial sweetener =	8 teaspoons sugar			
Lemon juice	1 teaspoon			
Lemon rind	a few gratings			
Flour, sifted	½ cup	48	6.4	.4
		48	27.4	15.4
Calories: 1 serving—50		5	3	2

Add salt to egg whites and beat until foamy. Add cream of tartar and continue beating until stiff, but not dry. Beat egg yolks until thick. Add artificial sweetener, lemon juice, and lemon rind while continuing to beat. Quickly and carefully fold egg yolks and flour which has been sifted several times into egg whites. Drop by spoonfuls into greased muffin pans or waxed paper baking cups. Bake at 350 degrees for 18 minutes.

Servings: 10
Exchange per serving: 1 fruit, ½ medium-fat meat

Low-Sugar Cupcakes

Ingredients	Measure	Carbohydrates (gm.)	Protein (gm.)	Fat (gm.)
Margarine	6 tablespoons			90
Egg	1		7	5
Milk, skim	½ cup	6	4	
Flour	1⅓ cups	128	17	
Vanilla	⅔ teaspoon			
Baking powder	3 teaspoons			
Artificial sweetener granulated	= ½ cup sugar			
		134	28	95
Calories: 1 serving—124		11	2	8

Cream margarine; add artificial sweetener and egg. Combine milk and vanilla. Sift together flour and baking powder. Add flour and milk mixtures alternately to margarine mixture. Spoon into 12 small muffin cups. Bake at 350 degrees for 25 to 30 minutes.

Servings: 12
Exchange per serving: ⅔ bread, 1½ fat

Aunt Tillie's Favorite Brownie Recipe

Ingredients	Measure	Carbohydrates (gm.)	Protein (gm.)	Fat (gm.)
Chocolate, semi-sweet	4 ounces	73.2	5.6	31.6
Milk, skim	½ cup	6	4	
Shortening	1 cup			240
Artificial sweetener, granulated =	2 cups sugar			
Eggs	4		28	20
Flour	1½ cups	144	19.2	
Salt	½ teaspoon			
Baking powder	1 teaspoon			
Vanilla	1 teaspoon			
		223.2	56.8	291.6
Calories: 1 serving—91		6	1	7

Melt chocolate in milk and let cool. Cream shortening; add artificial sweetener and eggs. Add chocolate mixture, dry ingredients, vanilla. Bake in greased 13×9×2-inch pan at 350 degrees for 30 minutes or until toothpick comes out dry when checked. Cut brownies when cool into 39 pieces, 3×1-inch.

If desired, add ½ cup chopped walnuts to batter or sprinkle on top before baking. This will then give ½ bread and 2 fat exchanges per brownie.

Servings: 39
Exchange per serving: ½ bread, 1½ fat

213

RECIPE FOR

Breakfast Coffee Cake

Ingredients	Measure	Carbohydrates (gm.)	Protein (gm.)	Fat (gm.)
Milk, skim	¼ cup	3	2	
Margarine	⅓ cup			79.5
Salt	1 teaspoon			
Artificial sweetener =	12 teaspoons sugar			
Yeast	2 packages			
Water, lukewarm	½ cup			
Eggs, beaten	2		14	10
Flour	3 cups	288	38	
Walnuts, chopped	⅓ cup			25
		291	54	114.5
Calories: 1 serving—269		36	6	13

Scald milk; add margarine, salt, and artificial sweetener; stir until margarine is melted. Cool to lukewarm. Dissolve yeast in warm water; add to the milk mixture. Add beaten eggs and flour, mix well and spoon into a greased 9-inch-square cake pan. Let rise, covered, in warm place until double in bulk. Scatter the chopped walnuts over top with light sprinkling of granulated artificial sweetener and cinnamon. Bake at 400 degrees for 20 minutes.

Servings: 9
Exchange per serving: 2 bread, 2½ fat

Cookies

Smackaroons

Ingredients	Measure	Car-bohy-drates (gm.)	Pro-tein (gm.)	Fat (gm.)
Egg whites	3	.6	9.9	
Double-acting baking powder	½ teaspoon			
Flour	2 tablespoons	12	2	
Artificial sweetener =	16 teaspoons sugar			
Almond extract	½ teaspoon			
Rice crispy cereal	2½ cups	50	6.7	
Coconut, unsweetened	¼ cup	12	3.6	32.4
		74.6	22.2	32.4
Calories: 4 cookies—109		12	4	5.2

Beat egg whites with baking powder until stiff but not dry. Blend in flour, artificial sweetener, almond extract, cereal, and coconut. Drop by rounded teaspoonfuls onto lightly greased cookie sheets. Bake at 350 degrees for 12 minutes.

Yield: 24 cookies
Exchange per serving: 4 cookies = 1 bread, 1 fat

Cinnamon Cookies

Ingredients	Measure		Car-bohy-drates (gm.)	Pro-tein (gm.)	Fat (gm.)
Margarine	5	tablespoons			75
Flour	1	cup	96	12.8	
Baking powder	½	teaspoon			
Cinnamon	1	teaspoon			
Salt		pinch			
Artificial sweetener	16 =	teaspoons sugar			
Vanilla	1	teaspoon			
Milk	1	tablespoon	.7	.5	
			96.7	13.3	75

Calories: 4 cookies—150   13   2   10

Cream margarine; blend in flour, baking powder, cinnamon, and salt. Mix artificial sweetener with vanilla and milk. Stir into flour mixture and mix thoroughly. Shape dough into 30 balls and place on cookie sheet. Flatten balls with fork dipped in cold water. Bake at 375 degrees for 15 minutes.

Yield: 30 cookies
Exchange per serving: 4 cookies = 1 bread, 2 fat

Pinwheel Cookies

Ingredients	Measure	Carbohydrates (gm.)	Protein (gm.)	Fat (gm.)
Flour	1½ cups	144	19.2	
Shortening	½ cup			120
Orange juice	¼ cup	5		
Margarine, soft	2 tablespoons			30
Nuts, chopped	⅓ cup			25
		149	19.2	175
Calories: 1 cookie—36		2	.3	3

Cut shortening into flour. Add juice and mix well. Divide into three portions and roll out each piece. Spread with soft margarine and sprinkle with mixture of nuts, cinnamon, and powdered artificial sweetener to taste. Roll and slice ¼ inch. Place cookies on sheet and bake at 450 degrees for 12 minutes.

The cookies can be spread with dietetic jelly instead of nut, cinnamon, and sugar mixture. In that case omit softened margarine. This will make each cookie 2 grams of fat instead of 2.9.

Yield: 60 cookies
Exchange per serving: 1 cookie = ⅛ bread, ½ fat

CHAPTER 19

Beverages

Tomato Tantalizer

Ingredients	Measure		Car- bohy- drates (gm.)	Pro- tein (gm.)	Fat (gm.)
Tomato juice	20 ounces		12.5	5	
Instant minced onion	1 tablespoon				
Artificial sweetener	½ teaspoon sugar	=			
Salt	½ teaspoon				
Worcestershire sauce	¼ teaspoon				
Tabasco	dash				

Combine all ingredients. Refrigerate. Serve in pre-chilled glasses. Sprinkle with coarse ground pepper.

Servings: 4
Exchange per serving: free

Ice Cream Float

Ingredients	Measure	Carbohydrates (gm.)	Protein (gm.)	Fat (gm.)
Vanilla ice cream	½ cup	15	2	10
Noncaloric carbonated beverage	8 ounces			
Calories: 1 serving—158		15	2	10

Put ice cream in glass and pour beverage on top.

Servings: 1
Exchange per serving: 1 bread, 2 fat

Milkshake

Ingredients	Measure	Carbohydrates (gm.)	Protein (gm.)	Fat (gm.)
Milk, skim	½ cup	6	4	
Artificial sweetener	= ½ teaspoon sugar			
Ice cube	1			
Vanilla	⅛ teaspoon			
Calories: 1 serving—40		6	4	

Place all ingredients in electric blender and blend until milkshake foams up and ice cube disappears.

In place of vanilla you can use almost any extract that pleases you—banana, orange, peppermint, etc.

Servings: 1
Exchange per serving: ½ milk

222

Appendixes

Brand-Name Products and Their Exchanges

BEVERAGES

GENERAL FOODS

Countrytime (8 ounces) lemonade, lemon-lime, pink lemonade	2 fruit
Tang (4 ounces) grape, grapefruit, orange	1½ fruit

LIPTON

Lemon Tree (8 ounces)	
Lemonade	2 fruit
Lemonade—sugar free	free
Iced Tea (8 ounces)	
Iced tea mix	1½ fruit
Iced tea mix—sugar free	free
Lemon-flavored (in cans)	2 fruit
Lemon-flavored—sugar free (in cans)	free

NESTLE'S

Hot cocoa mix (1 ounce)	1½ bread
Quik (¾ ounce)	
Chocolate	1 fruit, ½ bread
Strawberry	2 fruit

BREADS

QUAKER

Aunt Jemima Easy Mix
Coffee Cake (10.5 ounces;
⅛ portion of recipe)　　　2 bread, 1 fat

Aunt Jemima Easy Mix
Corn Bread (10 ounces;
⅙ portion of recipe)　　　2 bread, 1½ fat

Flako Corn Muffin Mix
(12 or 18 ounces; 1 corn
muffin)　　　　　　　　1½ bread, 1 fat

Flako Popover Mix (6
ounces; 1 popover)　　　　1½ bread, 1 fat

CAKES

QUAKER

Flako Cup Cake Mix
(11¾ ounces; 1 cupcake)　1½ bread, 1 fat

CEREALS, COLD

GENERAL FOODS

C. W. Post, with or without
raisins (¼ cup)　　　　　1½ bread, 1 fat

Post Alpha Bits (1 cup)　　1 bread, 1 fruit

Post 40% Bran Flakes
(⅔ cup)　　　　　　　　1½ bread

Post Grape Nuts (¼ cup)　1½ bread

Post Grape Nuts Flakes
(⅞ cup)　　　　　　　　1½ bread

Post Honeycomb (1⅓ cups)　1 bread, 1 fruit

225

Post Super Sugar Crisp
(⅞ cup)   1 bread, 1 fruit
Post Toasties Corn Flakes
(1¼ cups)   1 bread, 1 fruit

QUAKER

Cap'n Crunch (¾ cup)   1 bread, ¾ fruit, ½ fat
Cap'n Crunch with crunch-
berries (¾ cup)   1 bread, ¾ fruit, ½ fat
Corn Bran (⅔ cup)   1 bread, ¾ fruit
King Vitaman (¾ cup)   1 bread, ¾ fruit, ½ fat
Quisp (1⅙ cups)   1½ bread, ¾ fruit, ½ fat
Shredded Wheat
(2 biscuits)   1½ bread

RALSTON PURINA

Bran Chex (1 ounce; ⅔ cup) 1 bread, 1 fruit
Corn Chex (1 ounce; 1 cup) 1 bread, 1 fruit
Raisin Bran (1⅓ ounces;
¾ cup)   2 bread
Rice Chex (1 ounce; 1⅛
cups)   1 bread, 1 fruit
Wheat Chex (1 ounce;
⅔ cup)   1 bread, 1 fruit

CEREALS, HOT

QUAKER

Instant Oatmeal with
apples and cinnamon
(¾ cup cooked; 1 packet) 2 bread, ⅓ fat
Instant Oatmeal with bran
and raisins (¾ cup
cooked; 1 packet)   2 bread, ⅓ fat

Instant Oatmeal with cinnamon and spice (¾ cup cooked; 1 packet)	2 bread, ⅓ fat
Instant Oatmeal with maple and brown sugar (¾ cup cooked; 1 packet)	2 bread, ⅓ fat
Instant Oatmeal with raisins and spice (¾ cup cooked; 1 packet)	2 bread, ⅓ fat
Instant Oatmeal—regular (¾ cup cooked; 1 packet)	1 bread, ⅓ fat
Quaker Oats, quick or old-fashioned (⅓ cup uncooked; ⅔ cup cooked)	1 bread, ⅓ fat

CONDIMENTS

HEINZ

Hamburger relish (1 tablespoon)	1 vegetable
Hot dog relish (1 tablespoon)	1 vegetable
India relish (1 tablespoon)	1 vegetable
*Ketchup (hot) (1 tablespoon)	1 fruit
Mustard	free
Party relish (1 tablespoon)	1 fruit
Picalilli relish (1 tablespoon)	1 vegetable
*Tomato ketchup (1 tablespoon)	1 fruit
Unsweetened pickles	free
Vinegar	free

*Indicates products which, when used in a recipe, may be considered "free exchanges" with the approval of your diet counselor.

COOKIES
KEEBLER

Buttercup (2 cookies)	½ bread, ½ fat
Chocolate Fudge Sandwich (2 cookies)	1½ bread, 1½ fat
French Vanilla Creme (2 cookies)	1½ bread, 1½ fat
Pitter Patter (2 cookies)	1½ bread, 1½ fat
Vanilla Wafers (5 cookies)	1 bread, 1 fat

QUAKER

Chocolate Chip Cookie Mix (15 ounces; 2 cookies)	1 bread, 2 fat
Oatmeal Cookie Mix (18 ounces; 2 cookies)	1 bread, 1 fat
Peanut Butter Cookie Mix (15 ounces; 2 cookies)	1 bread, 2 fat

CRACKERS
KEEBLER

Snack Crackers (2 crackers) bacon, cheese, onion, pumpernickel, rye, sesame, wheat	¼ bread, ½ fat

DESSERTS
GELATIN

Dzerta (½ cup)	free
Jello (½ cup)	1 fruit

PUDDING

Dzerta (½ cup)   ½ fruit

Jello instant pudding and
    pie filling (½ cup) butter
    pecan, banana cream,
    butterscotch, chocolate,
    chocolate fudge, coconut
    cream, French vanilla,
    lemon, pineapple cream,
    pistachio, vanilla   2 bread, 1 fat

Jello pudding and pie filling
    (½ cup) butterscotch,
    chocolate, chocolate
    fudge, French vanilla,
    milk chocolate, vanilla   2 bread, 1 fat

FRENCH TOAST (see PANCAKES, WAFFLES, and FRENCH TOAST)

FRUIT, FROZEN

GENERAL FOODS

Birds Eye frozen fruit in
    quick-thaw pouch
    Mixed fruit (5 ounces)   3½ fruit
    Peaches (5 ounces)   3½ fruit
    Red raspberries (5
      ounces)   3½ fruit
    Strawberries (5 ounces)   3 fruit

LUNCHES, BOXED

LIPTON

Lite Lunch (7 ounces)

A la king	2 bread, ½ high-fat meat
Beef	1½ bread, ½ medium-fat meat
Chicken	1½ bread, ½ medium-fat meat
Garden vegetable	2 bread, ½ medium-fat meat
Noodles 'n cheese	2 bread, ½ high-fat meat, ½ fat
Oriental flavor	1½ bread, ½ medium-fat meat

LUNCHES, CANNED

FRANCO AMERICAN

Beef ravioli in meat sauce (7½ ounces)	1 vegetable, 2 bread, 1 low-fat meat
Beef Raviolios in meat sauce (7½ ounces)	1 vegetable, 2 bread, 1 low-fat meat
Elbow macaroni and cheese (7½ ounces)	2 bread, 1 fat
Macaroni and cheese (7½ ounces)	2 bread, 1 fat
Rotini and meatballs in tomato sauce (7½ ounces)	1 vegetable, 1½ bread, 1 low-fat meat, 1 fat
Rotini in tomato sauce (7½ ounces)	1 vegetable, 2 bread, 1 fat
Spaghetti in meat sauce (7½ ounces)	1 vegetable, 1 bread, 1 low-fat meat, 1½ fat
Spaghetti in tomato sauce with cheese (7½ ounces)	1 vegetable, 2 bread
Spaghetti with meatballs in tomato sauce (7½ ounces)	1 vegetable, 1 bread, 1 low-fat meat, 1 fat
SpaghettiOs in tomato and cheese sauce (7½ ounces)	2 bread

230

SpaghettiOs with little
meatballs in tomato
sauce (7½ ounces)   1 vegetable, 1 bread, 1 low-
fat meat, 1 fat

SpaghettiOs with sliced
franks in tomato sauce
(7½ ounces)   1 vegetable, 1½ bread, 2 fat

HEINZ

Beans and franks in
tomato sauce (7½ ounces)   1 vegetable, 2 bread, 1 low-
fat meat

Beans in tomato sauce,
vegetarian (8 ounces)   1 vegetable, 1 fruit, 2 bread

Beef goulash (7¼ ounces)   1 vegetable, 1 bread, 1 low-
fat meat, 2 fat

Beef stew (7¼ ounces)   1 vegetable, 1 bread, 1 low-
fat meat, 1 fat

Chicken stew with
dumplings (7¼ ounces)   1 vegetable, 1 bread, 1 low-
fat meat, 1 fat

Chili con carne with beans
(7½ ounces)   2 vegetable, 1 bread, 1 low-
fat meat, 3 fat

Chili and macaroni in
sauce (7½ ounces)   1½ bread, 1 low-fat meat,
2 fat

Macaroni and beef in
tomato sauce (7¼ ounces)   1 vegetable, 1 bread, 1 low-
fat meat, 1 fat

Macaroni in cheese sauce
(7½ ounces)   1½ bread, 1 low-fat meat,
½ fat

Noodles and tuna
(7½ ounces)   1 vegetable, 1 bread, 1 low-
fat meat

Noodles 'N' Chicken
(7¼ ounces)   1 bread, 1 low-fat meat,
1 fat

Noodles with beef and
sauce (7½ ounces)   1 bread, 1 low-fat meat,
½ fat

Pork 'N' Beans in tomato
sauce (8 ounces)   1 vegetable, 1 fruit, 2 bread,
1 low-fat meat

Spaghetti in tomato sauce
(cheese) (7½ ounces)   2 bread, ½ fat

Spaghetti with meat sauce (7¼ ounces)	1 vegetable, 1 bread, ½ low-fat meat, 1 fat
Spanish rice (7¼ ounces)	2 bread, 1 fat

LUNCHES, FROZEN

MORTON

Chili without beans (7½ ounces)	1 bread, 3 medium-fat meat, 1 fat
Meatball stew (8 ounces)	1 bread, 2 medium-fat meat, 1½ fat

SWANSON

Swanson Hungry Man
    Meat Pies (16 ounces)

Beef	1 vegetable, 4 bread, 3 low-fat meat, 7 fat
Chicken	1 vegetable, 4 bread, 3 low-fat meat, 7 fat
Sirloin burger	1 vegetable, 4 bread, 3 low-fat meat, 7 fat
Turkey	1 vegetable, 4 bread, 3 low-fat meat, 7 fat

Swanson Pies

Beef (8 ounces; 1 pie)	3 bread, 1 low-fat meat, 4 fat
Chicken (8 ounces; 1 pie)	3 bread, 1 low-fat meat, 4 fat
Turkey (8 ounces; 1 pie)	3 bread, 1 low-fat meat, 4 fat
Macaroni and cheese (7 ounces; 1 pie)	2 bread, 1 low-fat meat, 1 fat

Swanson Stews
(7½ ounces)

Beef — 1 vegetable, 1 bread, 1 low-fat meat, 1 fat

Chicken — 1 vegetable, 1 bread, 1 low-fat meat, 1 fat

Chicken and dumplings — 1 bread, 1 low-fat meat, 1 fat

PANCAKES, WAFFLES, AND FRENCH TOAST

GENERAL FOODS

Log Cabin Pancake and Waffle Mix (three 4-inch pancakes prepared with milk, egg, and shortening) — ¼ milk, 2 bread, 2 fat

QUAKER

Aunt Jemima Buckwheat Pancake and Waffle Mix (three 4-inch pancakes) — 1½ bread, 1½ fat

Aunt Jemima Buttermilk Pancake and Waffle Mix (three 4-inch pancakes) — 2½ bread, 2 fat

Aunt Jemima Complete Pancake and Waffle Mix (three 4-inch pancakes) — 2½ bread, ½ fat

Aunt Jemima French Toast, frozen (2 slices) — 2 bread, 1 fat

Aunt Jemima Jumbo Waffles, frozen (1 waffle) — 1 bread, ½ fat

Aunt Jemima Original Pancake and Waffle Mix (three 4-inch pancakes) — 2 bread, 1½ fat

Aunt Jemima Pancake
Batter (one 4-inch
pancake)   1 bread

PIE CRUST

JOHNSTON

Graham Cracker and
   Chocolate Ready Crusts
   (⅛ portion of recipe)   1 bread, 1 fat

QUAKER

Flako Pie Crust Mix
   (10 ounces; one 6–9-inch
   pie crust)   2 bread, 3 fat

POTATO PRODUCTS

FRENCH'S

Big Tate Potatoes
   au Gratin (½ cup)   1½ bread, 1 fat
Big Tate Potato Pancake
   Mix (3 ounces; three
   3-inch pancakes)   1 bread, 1 fat
Big Tate Scalloped Potatoes
   (½ cup)   1½ bread, 1 fat

GENERAL FOODS

Birds Eye frozen potatoes
   Cottage Fries
      (2.8 ounces)   1 bread, 1 fat
      Crinkle Cuts (3 ounces)   1 bread, 1 fat
      French Fries (3 ounces)   1 bread, 1 fat

Hash Browns (4 ounces)	1 bread
Hash Browns O'Brien (3 ounces)	1 bread
Shoestrings (3.3 ounces)	1 bread, 1 fat
Steak Fries (3 ounces)	1 bread, ½ fat
Tasti Fries (2.5 ounces)	1 bread, 1½ fat

SAUCES

FRENCH'S

Cheese sauce (package made with 1 cup whole milk—¼ cup)	½ milk, 1 fat
Stroganoff sauce (package made with 1⅓ cups whole milk—⅓ cup	⅔ milk, 1 fat
Sour cream sauce (package made with ½ cup whole milk—2½ tablespoons)	⅓ milk, 1 fat
Italian Style Spaghetti Sauce Mix (5 ounces; ⅝ cup)	1 bread, 1 fat

HEINZ

*Barbecue sauce (¼ cup)	1 bread
*Chili sauce (1 tablespoon)	1 fruit
*57 Sauce (1 tablespoon)	1 vegetable
*Savory sauce (1 tablespoon)	1 fruit
*Worcestershire Sauce (1 tablespoon)	1 vegetable

*Indicates products which, when used in a recipe, may be considered "free exchanges with the approval of your diet counselor.

HUNT WESSON

Prima Salsa Spaghetti Sauce (4 ounces) Regular, Mushroom, Meat	1½ bread, ½ fat
Stewed Tomatoes (4 ounces)	½ bread
Tomato Sauce (4 ounces) Regular, with bits, with mushrooms, with cheese	½ bread
Tomato Paste (3 ounces)	1 bread

MORTON

Barbecue sauce with beef for sloppy joes (5 ounces)	1½ bread, 2 medium-fat meat

SEASONINGS

FRENCH'S

Beef stew seasoning (1⅞ ounces)	½ fruit
Chili-O (1¾ ounces)	⅓ bread
Enchilada seasoning (1⅜ ounces)	⅓ bread
Ground beef seasoning with onion (1⅛ ounces)	½ bread
Hamburger seasoning (1 ounce)	⅓ bread
Meat marinade (1 ounce)	⅕ fruit
Meatball seasoning (1½ ounces)	½ bread
Meatloaf seasoning (1½ ounces)	⅓ bread

Sloppy joes seasoning (1½ ounces)	½ fruit
Taco seasoning (1¾ ounces)	⅓ bread

SOUPS

CAMPBELL'S

Campbell's Chunky Soups (½ can)	
Chunky beef	1 bread, 2 low-fat meat
Chunky chicken	1 vegetable, 1 bread, 2 low-fat meat
Chunky chicken vegetable	1½ bread, 1 low-fat meat, 1 fat
Chunky chicken with rice	1 bread, 2 low-fat meat
Chunky chili beef	2 bread, 2 low-fat meat
Chunky clam chowder (Manhattan)	1½ bread, 1 low-fat meat
Chunky minestrone	1½ bread, 1 low-fat meat
Chunky old-fashioned bean with ham	1 vegetable, 2 bread, 1 low-fat meat, 1 fat
Chunky old-fashioned vegetable beef	1 vegetable, 1 bread, 1 low-fat meat
Chunky sirloin burger	1 vegetable, 1 bread, 1 low-fat meat, 1 fat
Chunky split pea with ham	2 bread, 1 low-fat meat, ½ fat
Chunky steak and potato	1 bread, 2 low-fat meat
Chunky turkey	1 vegetable, 1 bread, 1 low-fat meat
Chunky vegetable	1 vegetable, 1 bread, 1 fat

Campbell's Soup for One
(1 Can)
- Bean, old-fashioned .... 2 bread, 1 fat
- Golden chicken and
  noodles .... 1 bread, 1 fat
- Tomato royale .... 2 bread, 1 fat
- Vegetable, old world .... 1 bread, 1 fat

Campbell's Soups (½ can)
- Asparagus, Cream of .... 1 bread, 1 fat
- Bean with bacon .... 2 bread, 1 low-fat meat,
  ½ fat
- Beef .... 1 bread, 1 low-fat meat
- Beef broth (bouillon) .... 1 vegetable
- Beef noodle .... 1 bread
- Black bean .... 1½ bread
- Celery, cream of .... ½ bread
- Cheddar cheese .... 1 milk, 3 fat
- Chicken alphabet .... 1 bread, 1 fat
- Chicken broth .... 1 low-fat meat
- Chicken, cream of .... ½ bread, 2 fat
- Chicken gumbo .... 1 bread
- Chicken 'n dumplings .... ½ bread, 1 low-fat meat,
  1 fat
- Chicken noodle .... 1 bread
- Chicken NoodleO's .... 1 bread
- Chicken and stars .... 1 bread
- Chicken vegetable .... 1 bread
- Chicken with rice .... 1 bread
- Chili beef .... 2 bread, 1 low-fat meat,
  ½ fat
- Clam chowder
  (Manhattan) .... 1 bread, ½ fat
- Consomme (beef) .... 1 low-fat meat
- Curly noodle with
  chicken .... 1 bread, ½ fat

238

Golden Vegetable NoodleO's	1 bread
Green pea	2 bread, 1 low-fat meat
Hot dog bean	2 bread, 1 low-fat meat, 1 fat
Meatball alphabet	1 bread, 1 low-fat meat, ½ fat
Minestrone	1 bread, ½ fat
Mushroom, cream of	1 bread, 2 fat
Mushroom, golden	1 bread, 1 fat
Noodles and ground beef	1 bread, 1 fat
Onion	1 bread
Pepper pot	1 bread, 1 low-fat meat, ½ fat
Scotch broth	1 bread, 1 fat
Split pea with ham and bacon	2 bread, 1 low-fat meat, ½ fat
Stockpot	1 bread, 1 low-fat meat
Tomato	1 vegetable, 1 bread
Tomato bisque	2 bread, ½ fat
Tomato rice, old-fashioned	2 bread
Turkey noodle	1 bread
Turkey vegetable	1 bread
Vegetable	1 vegetable, 1 bread
Vegetable beef	½ bread, 1 low-fat meat
Vegetable, old-fashioned	1 bread
Vegetarian vegetable	1 bread

LIPTON'S

Lipton Cup a Soup (6 ounces)	
Beef flavor noodle	½ bread
Chicken, cream of	½ bread, ½ fat
Chicken rice	½ bread

239

Chicken vegetable	½ bread
Green pea	1½ bread
Mushroom, cream of	½ bread, ½ fat
Onion	⅕ bread
Spring vegetable	½ bread
Tomato	1 bread
Vegetable, cream of	1 bread, ½ fat
Vegetable beef	½ bread

Lipton's Soups (8 ounces)

Beef mushroom	½ bread
Chicken noodle with chicken meat	½ bread, ⅓ meat
Chicken ripple noodle	1 bread, ⅓ meat
Country vegetable	1 bread
Giggle noodle	1 bread, ⅓ fat
Noodle with chicken broth	½ bread, ⅓ fat
Onion	½ bread
Onion mushroom	½ bread
Ring o Noodle	⅔ bread
Vegetable beef	⅔ bread

NESTLE'S

Souptime (1 envelope in 6 ounces of water)

Beef noodle	⅓ low-fat meat, ⅓ bread
Chicken, cream of	½ bread, 1 fat
Chicken noodle	⅓ low-fat meat, ⅓ bread
French onion	⅓ bread
Green pea	1 bread
Mushroom	½ bread, 1 fat
Tomato	1 bread
Vegetable, cream of	½ bread, 1 fat

STUFFING

GENERAL FOODS

Stove Top Stuffing Mix
  (with butter)
    Chicken (½ cup)   1½ bread, 2 fat
    Cornbread (½ cup)   1½ bread, 2 fat

WAFFLES (see PANCAKES, WAFFLES, AND FRENCH TOAST)

Carbohydrate, Protein, Fat, and Calorie Counts for Various Cooking Ingredients

	Carbo-hydrates (gm.)	Pro-tein (gm.)	Fat (gm.)	Calories
Bisquick (1 cup)	76	9.5	14.5	472.5
Brown sugar (1 tablespoon)	13			52
Chocolate				
Baker's German sweet (4½ square; 1 ounce)	16.6	1.1	10.4	162.6
Baker's semi-sweet chips (1 ounce)	18.3	1.4	7.9	147.9
Baker's unsweetened (1 square; 1 ounce)	8	4	15.1	183.9
Nestle's Choco-Bake (1 ounce)	12	2	14	170

Food				
Nestle's milk chocolate morsels (1 ounce)	17	2	9	150
Coconut, unsweetened (¼ cup)	12	3.6	32.4	354
Cornstarch (2 tablespoons)	15	2		68
Dessert toppings				
Cool Whip (5 tablespoons)	5		5	70
Dream Whip (1 tablespoon)	.6	.3	.6	9
Dzerta low calorie whipped topping mix (1 tablespoon)			1	8
Flour (white commercial)				
1 cup	96	12.8		435
½ cup	48	6.4		217
1 tablespoon	6	.1		27
Gelatin, unflavored (1 envelope)		7		28
Graham cracker crust— Johnston's				
whole	117	9.1	36	828.4
⅛ pie crust	15	1.1	4.6	104.9
Graham crackers (1 cup, crushed—12 crackers)	90	12		408
Ground meat (after cooking)				
1 pound		84	96	1200
½ pound		42	48	600
¼ pound		21	24	300
Ketchup (1 tablespoon)	4.9	.4		21.2
Macaroni; uncooked (1 ounce)	15	2		68
Marshmallows (8; 1 ounce)	23	1		96
Orange juice frozen concentrate (1 ounce)	10			40

Tomato paste (1 ounce)	7	2		36
Tomato sauce (2 ounces)	7	2		36
Walnuts, chopped (⅓ cup)	5		5	70

How to Calculate Favorite Recipes

On a blank sheet, list each ingredient, the amount to be used for the recipe and, in the proper columns, the carbohydrate, protein, and fat count of this amount in grams. (This can be found for most items in the beginning of each exchange category or in the listing of products in the Appendix.)

Add up the totals in each column and divide by the number of servings. This will tell you the amount of carbohydrate, protein, and fat for each serving. Using the chart below, calculate how many of each exchange the serving will cover.

Figures are in grams per exchange.

	Carbo-hydrates (gm.)	Pro-tein (gm.)	Fat (gm.)	Calories
Bread	15	2		70
Fat			5	45
Fruit	10			40
Meat				
Low-fat		7	3	55
Medium-fat		7	5.5	77.5
High-fat		7	8	100
Milk	12	8		80
Vegetable	5	2		25

Weights and Measures

1 teaspoon	⅓ tablespoon
1 tablespoon	3 tablespoons
¼ cup	4 tablespoons
½ cup	5⅓ tablespoons
1 cup (liquid)—8 ounces	16 tablespoons
1 ounce (liquid)	2 tablespoons
1 ounce (dry measure)	¹⁄₁₆ pound
1 pint	2 cups
1 quart	2 pints
1 gallon	4 quarts
1 gill	½ cup
1 bushel	4 pecks

SOURCES

American Diabetes Association, Incorporated
2 Park Avenue, 16th Floor
New York, New York   10016

Campbell Soup Company
Campbell Place
Camden, New Jersey   08101

R. T. French Company
One Mustard Street
Post Office Box 23450
Rochester, New York   14692

General Foods
250 North Street
White Plains, New York   10625

H. J. Heinz Company
Post Office Box 57
Pittsburgh, Pennsylvania   15230

Hunt Wesson Foods, Incorporated
1645 West Valencia Drive
Fullerton, California   92634

Keebler Company
One Hollow Tree Lane
Elmhurst, Illinois   60126

Thomas J. Lipton, Incorporated
800 Sylvan Avenue
Englewood Cliffs, New Jersey   07632

The Nestle Company, Incorporated
White Plains, New York   10605

The Quaker Oats Company
Merchandise Mart Plaza
Chicago, Illinois   60654

Ralston Purina Company
Checkerboard Square
St. Louis, Missouri   63185

INDEX

249

253